Delay, Don't Deny

Living an Intermittent Fasting Lifestyle

Gin Stephens

Author's Note
September 2018

People have told me that reading *Delay, Don't Deny* is like having a conversation with a friend...a friend you can trust...a friend who is apparently AWFUL at finding typos within her own writing.

"Typos are everywhere." This is one of my husband's favorite sayings...and, he's right. Since I first released *Delay, Don't Deny* in 2016, a number of typos were discovered within the book. This is a new-and-hopefully-typo-free version. But, then again, I think back to what my husband says. So, please enjoy this (probably? maybe? hopefully?) typo-free edition of *Delay, Don't Deny*. (And, if you find one, that's just the one I put in on purpose to see if you were paying attention.)

Also by Gin Stephens:

Feast Without Fear:
Food and the Delay, Don't Deny Lifestyle

Delay, Don't Deny LIFE Journal:
Charting Your Intermittent Fasting Lifestyle

Delay, Don't Deny Digging Deeper:
Advancing Your Intermittent Fasting Lifestyle

These books are available through most online book and e-book retailers.

Visit
www.ginstephens.com
for blog posts, intermittent fasting success stories, and more

----

Subscribe to *The Intermittent Fasting Podcast*!
Go to
www.ifpodcast.com
to learn more

DEDICATION

This book is dedicated to my husband, Chad Stephens. Thank you for loving me through thick and thin: literally. You have been incredibly patient with all of my crazy diet schemes over the years, and I am grateful.

This photo was taken in 1991, right before our wedding day.
We were clearly babies: I was 21, and he was 20.
And just like most women, I look at this photo and notice how chubby I was.
I don't notice how sweet it is: I immediately criticize my appearance.
I am also very critical of the outfit, but at the time, I am sure I liked it.

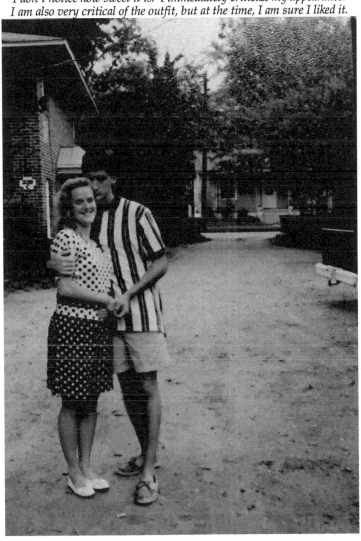

Table of Contents

Foreword

Are you there, Hippocrates? It's me, Ken.

Remember that oath I took on the day I earned my M.D.? Well, 20 years later it seems I may not have been quite as faithful as I once promised. You remember how I vowed:

> to *"do no harm" and to "prevent*
> *disease whenever I can, for*
> *prevention is preferable to cure"?*

I've always had the best intentions. I didn't purposely mislead my patients when I lectured them about their eating - I just didn't know better! It was once a secret that we physicians are not trained in nutrition; we are experts in pathology and pharmacology. Yet I am asked many times each day how to "fix obesity."

But I'm doing better. I'm slowly making up for the years of lecturing my patients that they should eat 3 "well-balanced" meals each day, with a few low-fat snacks thrown in between (you know, to keep the metabolism revved up). Then, I was getting closer when I advocated a lower carb / *higher fat* diet for helping diabetes - but not everyone is a diabetic. Measuring early morning insulin levels on my "difficult" patients got me closer still, but as far as what (*or WHEN?*) to eat, I seemed to be getting mixed results at best.

Despite *endless advice on different diets*, it seems like eventually doctors simply end up prescribing medications for cholesterol and high blood pressure. So are we any better off with this professional advice? Our country is plagued with record high levels of obesity, type 2 diabetes, hypertension, arthritis, inflammatory diseases, irritable

1

bowel, fibromyalgia, mood-disorders, and attention-deficit-disorders: it feels like this is a "new normal."

Every day there's another new pharmaceutical commercial. This can't be right. What is going on here?

This book tells it like it is: the problem for millions of people can be blamed on a society that has been transformed - we are living in an obesogenic environment. Your chance of staying fit & healthy without a clear strategy is near zero. Why do you think every casino has an all-you-can-eat-buffet? Think about it. Your body is a machine, controlled by a series of hormones that control your appetite and your self-control. Do you *need* to eat 6 times a day to thrive? Do you *need* diet soft drinks to be happy? *Really?* Who's in control here? Who's been programming these feelings/emotions?

Feeding your body (your machine) is a game of big business. Treating the diseases associated with your obese body (your broken machine) is also big business. Information on "nutrition" has to be disseminated (read, paid) by someone, right? Take every study you read on Facebook with a major grain of salt. Come to think of it, after reading this book you'll know you can stop worrying about salt too! Keep an open mind with this - there is some very powerful knowledge in here! But it goes against the grain, against the norm, against what is commonly believed… *remember that.*

Gin Stephens has knocked one out of the park with *Delay, Don't Deny*. As you read this (several times), you'll find yourself getting lost in "a conversation" you're having with Gin. She's fun, and easy to talk to, but she dishes out some tough love as well! There's no quick gimmick in here, but a promise of better health awaits those who follow through.

My single hope is that you take your time and truly appreciate the science she covers here. Intermittent fasting is the real deal. It has dozens of well-funded, well-executed scientific studies. The protocols she describes are safe, effective, and scientifically valid. Just ask any of the thousands of followers on her Facebook support group. (Hint: search the book title on Facebook - do it now!)

Best of all, she is describing a way out of the game forever. It's getting old, and you're not getting any younger! This truly is a way to change your lifestyle so your body's health improves each day, month after month: less body fat, improved metabolism, reduced dependence on medications, improved blood pressure, normalization of blood sugar... not to mention improved mental clarity, self-discipline, and self-confidence. Have I mentioned that fasting has anti-aging benefits and probably improves your life expectancy? Not bad, huh?

The world's a different place than when the first Hippocratic oath was written ~ 400 BCE. Heck, the information in this book wasn't widely known 10 years ago! It truly is an exciting time for us scientists who seek better health through nutrition. You will soon become your own experiment of one, and you have an entire legion of like-minded pioneers supporting you. Congratulate yourself on becoming part of a real movement.

So I'll try a little harder to adhere to my promises over the next 20 years. No more canned responses when my next patient comes to me desperate for answers on how to lose weight. I'll just have them enjoy a "conversation with Gin," and then support them on their lifetime journey of experimenting and researching the various intermittent fasting options that work for them.

Kenneth Power, MD, CFPC
Dec. 2016

Disclaimer

This book is not a substitute for medical advice. All information and tools presented within this text are intended for motivational purposes. Any health, diet, or exercise advice shared here is <u>not</u> intended as medical diagnosis or treatment. If you think you have any type of medical condition, you must seek professional advice, even if you believe it may be due to diet, food, or exercise. You should always consult a qualified practitioner before using any dietary, exercise, or health advice from this text.

Introduction

About me, and what to expect from this book

Okay, you caught me. I am not a medical doctor, and I am not a nutritionist. You may be asking yourself why you should listen to a regular person like me when it comes to dietary advice. Of course, you should not take medical advice from random people that you don't know, and that includes me. Always check with your favorite trusted medical professionals when making decisions that could affect your health. If you have a medical condition, you absolutely have to talk to your physician before changing your lifestyle. Nothing in this book should be considered by you to be medical advice from me. Go read the disclaimer if you haven't read it already.

Now that I've gotten that out of the way, I want to tell you a little bit about who I am. I am a 47-year-old mother of 2 teenage sons. I have been married to my patient husband for over 25 years, and, as I mentioned on the dedication page, he has literally loved me through thick and thin. (Some years were thicker than others...) Like many of you, I have struggled with my weight for years—decades even—and I have tried so many different ways to lose weight. If you want to read my whole convoluted story, turn right to Appendix A for my dieting and weight loss story. I have laid it out there for you, and you may have a diet history just as crazy as mine.

No, I am not a medical doctor. I do, however, have a doctorate in Gifted and Talented Education, and I was at one time a member of Mensa. (I am actually a Mensa dropout. Oops.) I don't tell you this to brag about how smart I am, but to let you know that I am able to at least get a paper successfully past a dissertation committee and pass an intelligence test. Hopefully, that will give me some credibility. If that doesn't, maybe the fact that I have lost 80+ pounds and kept it off for 2 years now (as of early 2017) should do it.

Both of these photos show me with my sons. The photo on the left is from April of 2014. I weighed about 210 pounds. This photo got my attention, as I couldn't believe that was me. Can you say "denial"? The second photo is from December of 2016, after I lost 80+ pounds. I'm going to start telling people I am their sister, because I don't know how those grown men can possibly be my babies.

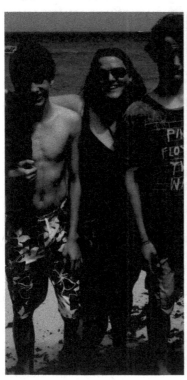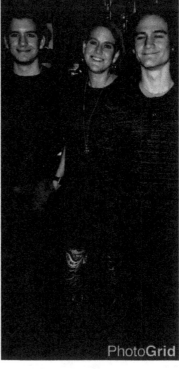

If it makes you feel better, you can call me Dr. Stephens. My elementary gifted students call me that all day, and I will definitely answer to it. Or, you can just call me Gin, and I will be your Gin-spiration throughout this book. Think of me as a trusted friend, and imagine that we are having a casual conversation about how you can approach the business of weight loss and eventual weight maintenance.

The goal of this book is to share some of the latest thinking about the weight loss strategy known as intermittent fasting. I will tell you my story and point you towards some fantastic books that WERE written by researchers and medical doctors. You do not have to take it from me—after reading my story, you can go straight to the books written by actual medical professionals and read what they have to say. You'll find an annotated bibliography of resources in Appendix C.

I want to warn you right up front: the writing style of this book is going to be casual. I am going to refer to sources, but not in a formal way. Many of the books I will point you to in the annotated bibliography DO have comprehensive reference lists, and if you love to read scientific papers, you will find complete lists of suggested scientific sources in those reference sections. Throughout this book, I will be paraphrasing and summarizing information based on my understanding of the issues, but to gain a deeper understanding, I highly suggest that you dig deeper using the resources I recommend. I will mention some scientific thinking, but I am not going to be overly science-y (and I might even make up some words, as I just did there with science-y).

Ready to get started? Keep reading!

Chapter 1

All of the diets work and none of them work

Diets. Even the word sounds restrictive. How many times have you read a new diet book, and when you started you were full of enthusiasm for the plan? WOW! Everything makes so much sense. The science seems to be there. You can literally eat WHATEVER YOU WANT and the pounds will fall right off.

Then you read a little more of the book. Hmmmm. It's not really "whatever you want." You have to limit carbs. Or meat. Or fat. Or sugar. Or things that start with the letter S. (That's a real book, people.) But it is okay, because there are so many wonderful things that you CAN eat that you are not even going to MISS carbs/meat/fat/sugar/S-words! Trust me! Life is delicious and satisfying, and you won't miss it at all! (That is the biggest lie ever, by the way. After the first week or two, you WILL miss carbs/meat/fat/sugar/S-words so much that you dive headfirst into a vat of the forbidden foods and there's the end of that diet. Again. Oops.)

Even though my degree is not in nutrition or medicine, over the years, I have read everything about weight loss that I could get my hands on. Each time I read a new weight loss book, I would try the plan out and see if it worked for me. (Unless I knew within the first few pages that it was going to be too hard because of my inherent laziness, in which case I would just stop reading and chalk that book purchase up as another mistake. Amazon loves me.) I have read many excellent books (and also some that are worthless), and I probably have read more about nutrition than many physicians. Do you know what is funny, though? So much of what I have read WAS written by doctors, and each of the books directly contradicts at least one of the other books. You know I am right. It is incredibly frustrating to see how much contradictory information is out there.

Many of the diet books promoted plans that were overly complicated, and I just couldn't keep up with the rigorous demands and rules. Have you tried the one where you pack up your food in dozens of tiny containers so you can snack on them all day long just to keep your metabolism stoked? Me, too! Who has time to prep all of that food? I certainly do not. How about the diet books where you don't eat any carbs, ever? Of course, I am again talking about food that you have to spend the weekend cooking and packing up, because the food you can find in the real world doesn't meet your stringent carb count criteria. I've done that, and it wore me out. What about the plan where you can only eat "clean" foods and follow certain rules about what is allowed? "I'm sorry, was that carrot organically farmed by Tibetan Monks? If not, then I will not be eating it, Thankyouverymuch." The problem with all of these special food plans is that I don't have time (or the willpower) to keep up any kind of rigorous schedule where I have to work hard to always have a certain kind of food with me, or to have certain foods that are eternally off limits. Like you, some days I have to work until 6 p.m., and then I may want to eat dinner that I can pick up on the way home. There is no drive through that dispenses fancy meals that meet all of the dietary restrictions that go with each wacky diet I tried, so eventually, each plan was destined to failure for me.

What about the magical supplements that you can buy that will magically allow you to magically lose the fat from your trouble areas, magically? Been there, bought those. I used to watch Dr. Oz every day, and I would be glued to the LATEST WEIGHT LOSS MIRACLE! segment every time, knowing that, YES! This is my problem! I am deficient in this herb that is grown in the Amazonian Rain Forest, and once I start taking this miracle cure I will be THIN! The fat will melt off of my body! I would order each miracle supplement and then start the regimen that would allow me to effortlessly drop the fat. Usually, you had to take 3 capsules of this AMAZING herb 20 minutes before each meal, and then EAT WHATEVER YOU WANT and watch the pounds melt off. Again, compliance was a problem for me. I would forget to take the capsules, or I wouldn't have them with me, and eventually, I would just stop taking them and add them to the drawer of failed miracle supplements. Thank the Lord I finally came to my senses and stopped DVR'ing Dr. Oz. These days I don't even look directly at magazine covers if he is on them. Dr. Oz, you cost me a fortune.

This is why all diets work, and no diets work. We can follow a crazy restrictive regimen for a while, and we may even lose some weight, but eventually, you are going to want to eat pizza or cake or Thanksgiving dinner. These "diet" plans are just not sustainable long-term. The good news is that with intermittent fasting, you don't have to follow a crazy diet. You can eat the foods you want to eat, and you can lose the guilt.

After years of struggling, and learning that I am not going to follow a traditional diet or keep up a difficult schedule of supplementation, I FINALLY feel a confident sense of peace that I have found the key to permanent weight loss. Over a 10-month period, I lost 75 pounds (which has turned into 80+...yes, I continue to lose fat slowly while in maintenance), using techniques that fit in nicely with my overall eating preferences. The best news is that my new eating style doesn't require me to make elaborate plans about what I will be eating, and there is actually a wealth of cutting-edge research that shows that my new eating style is healthier than traditional diets. I am thrilled to report that I have been maintaining this weight loss for about 2 years now (and, in fact, I have gotten even leaner over the past year without even trying). This is almost unheard of in today's world where statistics show that the vast majority of people who lose weight gain it all back. (I have seen estimates that only about 5% of people are able to keep off the weight long term. That sure is depressing, isn't it?)

So—if you are sick of trying to find the perfect diet for you, and instead want to find a lifestyle that you can tailor to suit your eating preferences, you are in the right place. Intermittent fasting is not only free, but it also allows you to eat whatever you want. The solution is literally in the title of this book: you will learn to DELAY eating, rather than to DENY yourself.

Chapter 2

The obesity epidemic—Why are we so fat?

It's very simple in theory. At any given moment, you can either be burning fuel from the last meal you ate, or you can be burning stored fat from your body. When you reach a point of balance—where the amount of food you eat in a day perfectly matches the amount of fuel your body needs to burn in a day—you have weight maintenance. If you are eating more than your body can burn, you have fat gain. If you burn more than you store, you have fat loss. Clearly, that is the goal for anyone who is attempting to lose weight. You want to burn more fat than your body can store.

HOW to actually do that is the big question that haunted me for years. You can probably relate. If it were easy to figure out, we would all be slim. (*Gin looks around. Nope, we are not all slim yet.*) In fact, data shows that Americans are getting bigger and bigger over time.

WHY can't we figure this out, if it is as simple as just eating less food?

There are many answers to this question, depending upon who you ask. If you ask almost anyone you meet, the answer would be that we eat too much and don't move enough. That's the conventional "eat less, move more" strategy. It sounds so simple, doesn't it? All we have to do is eat less, and move more, and we will be thin and healthy.

We have all heard this advice and tried to follow it, and it is not quite so simple in practice. Why is that?

Well then, it must be because we lack self-control. We all WANT to eat less and move more, which we have heard is the only way to lose weight. So—if we are unsuccessful, it must be because we are spineless and gluttons and weak human beings. Good news! You are not a spineless glutton. I don't even know you, and I know that to be true. There is a lot going on in your body that is out of your control. If you try to eat less over a long period of time, then certain hunger hormones are activated that make you want to eat and eat and eat. It's because your body LOVES you, and doesn't want you to starve to death! Your body doesn't know that you are purposefully restricting your food intake, and it thinks you must be in some sort of terrible famine. The hunger hormones cause you to seek out whatever food you can find, and that's when you end up standing at the refrigerator door eating anything you can shove into your mouth. Been there, done that. That's the moment when you feel like a weak failure with no self-control. When you realize WHY you feel that way—because it is your body trying to keep you alive—you can cut yourself some slack.

Others would say that we are fat because portions are bigger. Well, I'm pretty sure that we do expect bigger portions these days, whether we are eating at home or at a restaurant. All I have to do is think about my grandmother's generation and how they ate. When she died, I inherited her fine china. You should see how small the serving bowls and serving platters are! The serving bowls are not much bigger than the cereal bowls you can buy now at most stores. And the set has tiny little coffee cups and saucers! There were no giant coffee mugs or huge travel tumblers back then for us to fill with creamy coffee goodness and drink on the go. No, they would sit and drink their tiny little cups of coffee and then be done with it. The set also comes with a cream and sugar service, and the cream pitcher holds less cream than I would use for one cup of coffee. So, there is an element of truth in the idea of bigger portions. Maybe if we had never started eating huge meals, we wouldn't see such an obesity epidemic. I have a feeling, though, that big portions are here to stay.

I have also heard people blame the fact that we eat out more. Just look at the number of restaurants all around us, particularly fast food restaurants. Not only are there more and more restaurant options to choose from, but we are busy. Many families have either one single working parent or two parents who are both working. When you are working all day long, it can be hard to find the energy to come home and put a balanced meal on the table. It is SO much easier to pick up something on the way home, or rely on packaged foods from the supermarket. Unfortunately, many things we can pick up or prepare in a hurry are devoid of nutrients and not the highest quality.

One other thought is that our food supply is different now. In some areas, the soil has been depleted of nutrients due to years of farming, and we are genetically modifying many of our crops. We add corn syrup to almost everything, and there are artificial flavors, colors, sweeteners, and preservatives in many store-bought foods. Grocery store food is certainly different than what our great-grandparents ate. One popular diet book tells us that even wheat available today is different than it used to be. So why does all of this matter? I've read the theory that our bodies don't recognize these artificially grown and developed items as "food." (Doritos, though delicious, are not picked from a Dorito bush.) Because of that, our bodies are always in search of nutrients, which makes us hungrier. We eat and eat, yet never feel satisfied.

So: our portions are bigger, we eat out more, we reach for convenience foods, and our food supply has changed. Our hunger hormones are on overdrive because we have tried (unsuccessfully) to restrict what we are eating and we are eating processed junk. I do think that all of these factors work together to make it harder for us to lose weight; however, I think there is an even bigger culprit, and this is the piece of the puzzle I was always missing when I tried to change WHAT I was eating. The problem is meal frequency: we are constantly in a fed state, and never get a chance to access our stored fat. By changing WHEN I was eating, I was able to lose weight while worrying less about WHAT I was eating.

Why are we constantly in a fed state? Think about it for a minute. What is the latest dietary advice? If you said, "eat frequent and small meals throughout the day to fuel your metabolism," then you are right on target. This very advice is why we are having so much trouble losing weight. Are there people who can eat frequent small meals during the day and lose weight? Of course, there are! I am not one of them, however, and if you have struggled with your weight, you probably aren't one of them, either.

In this book, you will learn how to FINALLY enter a fat burning state every day of your life, so that you can access the fat you have stored on your body. The best news of all? You can do it eating the foods you love. Again, remember the name of the book: *Delay, Don't Deny!*

Chapter 3

The problem with calories

As I mentioned in the beginning of the book, I am going to summarize what I have learned about how the body works. Remember that I am not a medical doctor or a nutritionist, and keep that in mind as you read. Also, remember that nothing I am discussing should be considered to be specific medical advice from me to you. There are fantastic books written by actual medical doctors and experts in the field (see the annotated bibliography, located in Appendix C, for my recommendations) that you can (and should) refer to in order to learn more about these topics. I am going to hit the highlights so that you have a basic understanding of what is going on in our bodies. Perhaps my analogies or explanations will be over-simplified in places; remember, I am an elementary teacher, so I spend my whole day simplifying complex things so that young kids will understand them.

Now, for some science.

Conventional diet advice tells you that you have to restrict calories to lose weight. Everyone knows this. As I mentioned in the last chapter, it is simple: you must burn more energy than you take in if you want to lose weight.

Scientists have figured out a way to measure the amount of energy in various foods in a lab, and they call the energy "calories." Back in the day, our great-grandparents didn't know what calories were. Somehow, they were able to eat appropriate amounts of food, and it was rare to see an obese person back then. How did they do it without counting calories, when they didn't even know what calories were?

By now, though, we've all heard of calories, and most of us have tried to count them at one time or another. Scientists have shown that the calorie calculations of various foods are consistent over time...in a lab. Unfortunately (or fortunately), your body is not a lab. Think about it: do you really believe that you could eat 1200 calories of jelly beans and have the same outcome as if you eat 1200 calories of raw vegetables? Spoiler alert: you can't. At least, not long term.

The theory that our bodies work like a calorie calculator can be called "calories in/calories out," and I am going to refer to it using the common abbreviation: CI/CO. My very favorite weight loss expert, Dr. Jason Fung, has named it the "Calorie Restriction as Primary" theory, which he refers to as the CRaP theory. This makes me giggle every time I read it. I have included his fantastic book, *The Obesity Code*, in the annotated bibliography (located in Appendix C). He also has a blog at the Intensive Dietary Management website, and I highly recommend it. I have learned a lot from his book and blog. Another fantastic book that debunks the CI/CO theory is *Good Calories, Bad Calories*, by Gary Taubes.

So, why is CI/CO CRaP when the theory sounds so good and is so widely circulated as the only way to lose weight effectively? It's because it doesn't work for us long term. You may have tried a calorie counting diet before. You started counting your calories diligently, you stuck to your plan, and, YES! You were rewarded with weight loss. Week after week, your weight went down, until you reached your goal weight. Once you got to your goal weight, you were able to effortlessly maintain your ideal weight by continuing to count calories, and The End, you lived happily ever after in your goal wardrobe.

Is that how it worked for you? No? Me neither.

Why is that? Let's take a lesson from the hit television show *The Biggest Loser*. In this reality show, the contestants lose truly amazing amounts of weight each week by following the magic formula of CI/CO. They reduce their "calories in" dramatically, and amp-up their "calories out" through so much physical exertion that they often become physically ill right on television. Now, that's entertainment! For the final episode of the year, the contestants return to reveal their final transformations. These are truly inspiring stories of people who have worked harder than they have ever worked in their lives to conquer the obesity demons that they have struggled with for so long. They look fantastic, and the audience is inspired.

Let me share their dirty little secret with you: their long-term results are abysmal. Horrific. Shocking. The contestants have very little long-term success, and notice that they have never had a reunion show where everyone is slim and fit. I have a link to share with you:

https://www.ncbi.nlm.nih.gov/pubmed/27136388

That link will take you to the abstract of a study conducted in 2016 called "Persistent Metabolic Adaptation 6 Years After 'The Biggest Loser' Competition." The title of the study tells it all. The contestants featured in the show suffered from something called "persistent metabolic adaptation" after their amazing transformations. This means that their metabolisms had slowed down more than would be expected. This study showed that the period of prolonged calorie restriction—their CI/CO marathon—had an adverse effect that cost the participants 500 calories per day. They had to eat 500 FEWER CALORIES for their new weights than calculations based on body size alone would predict, just to maintain their new weights.

Here is an example of what that would look like in the real world. If we perform standard metabolic calculations on a hypothetical 5′ 5″ 40-year-old woman who weighs 125 pounds and is "moderately active," the calculator tells us that she is supposed to burn about 2036 calories per day, based on size and activity level. What the Biggest Loser study found is that instead of burning the expected number of calories, the participants' average metabolic rate was decreased by approximately 500 calories. In our hypothetical example, that would be a metabolic rate of 1536 calories to maintain her weight (instead of the expected 2036). Before the show, these contestants had normal metabolic rates, as calculated for their sizes. As they lost weight, their bodies slowed their metabolisms to compensate. But after the show, their metabolisms never recovered. They never again burned the "expected" number of calories for their size.

Dr. Fung does a phenomenal job explaining why this happens in his blog at Intensive Dietary Management. I encourage you to go there and read it. To simplify it for you here, all you need to really know is that the body did just what it was designed to do. Metabolic rate slowed down to protect the contestants. When the body perceives prolonged calorie restriction, it will slow down your metabolism as a protective measure. Research shows this clearly, as illustrated in the Biggest Loser study.

So—are we doomed for failure? I know that was the tone of all of the news reports that came out after this study was released. And, if counting calories was the only tool we had for weight loss, then I would agree—why bother, if we are doomed to a life of constant deprivation? Fortunately, as I said, the body is not a calorie calculator. Instead, the body works based on hormonal signals and responses that happen behind the scenes. Instead of worrying about how many calories you are eating, what you really need to worry about is how much insulin your body is releasing during the day. In the next chapter, you'll learn about why that is so important.

Chapter 4

Insulin: The key to unlocking your fat stores

What is insulin and why is it important? You may only know of insulin as something prescribed to diabetics, and you may give little thought to how it works in a normal body.

To oversimplify for the sake of basic understanding, every time you eat or drink certain things, your body releases insulin in response (unless you are a type 1 diabetic).   Insulin's job is to help your body regulate your blood glucose. When you eat, your blood sugar is available to be either burned as energy or stored in the body as glycogen—think of it as quick energy for later that is easily accessible. Any that is not burned as energy or stored as glycogen is turned into fat. Insulin is the conductor of the blood sugar train. We need insulin for this process to occur!

This is why type 1 diabetics rely on insulin injections that they must carefully adjust to match everything they consume. Without insulin, they are unable to properly utilize their blood glucose, which leads to dramatic weight loss. In 150 AD, the Greek physician Arateus described the condition as "the melting down of flesh and limbs into urine." The early tests for diabetes involved tasting the urine, and the unlucky physician was rewarded by a taste of sweetly flavored urine. (I know modern doctors are happy that we have new diagnostic techniques.) Without insulin, no matter how much diabetics eat, they continue to lose weight to an unhealthy degree. There goes the CI/CO theory! It's not a lack of "calories" that are causing them to lose weight; it's a lack of insulin!

Insulin also holds the key to the fat that is already in your fat cells. When you have a lot of insulin circulating throughout your body, your body is not going to be able to easily access your stored fat. It's a fat STORING hormone, after all. If you remember this piece of the puzzle, you are on your way to solving your fat burning problem.

Lots of circulating insulin = efficient fat storage and very little fat burning.

One other problem with high insulin levels is that our bodies adjust over time to elevated levels of insulin, which leads to more insulin being released, which leads to even higher levels of circulating insulin. This is known as insulin resistance. When you develop insulin resistance, your body has to release more and more insulin just to do the job, because, in theory, your body has "stopped listening" to the normal amount of insulin. It's like a class of kids with a teacher who yells at them all of the time. Eventually, the kids stop listening, and they tune out the yelling. So the teacher yells MORE! It's a vicious cycle. The kids have developed "yelling resistance," so the teacher has to yell more frequently to try to get their attention.

Remember—the more insulin you have circulating, the easier it is for you to store fat and the harder it is for you to access stored fat. Your body becomes very efficient at stuffing all of your fat cells full of energy and isn't accessing any of your stored fat for energy. This leads to excessive hunger, because the foods you eat get stored away as fat so readily. (Thanks, insulin!) So now you are eating more, storing it away efficiently as fat, and you are constantly ravenous.

There is a lot of complexity to the process, and rather than try to explain all of it (and risk making huge errors), I

24

am going to refer you to the excellent explanations written in the various books listed in Appendix C. Dr. Fung explains it beautifully in *The Obesity Code*. There are also other hormones that have roles in the process, such as leptin and ghrelin. I'll mention those appetite control hormones in a bit more depth later. If you love science and want to understand more about what is happening with all of these hormones, please take some time to research and learn more. It's fascinating stuff! (And, it makes you wonder why ANYONE can believe in straight up CI/CO anymore...)

I may have just oversimplified the complex processes at play, but what you need to take away from this chapter is this: by focusing on calories, many of us have missed one of the main drivers of the obesity crisis, and that is insulin. In order to lose weight successfully, you need to figure out how to lower your insulin levels so that your body can access your stored fat effectively. Rather than counting calories and tanking our metabolisms, as we saw with the Biggest Losers, we need to access our stored fat and keep our metabolisms working at high speed so that we can maintain our weight loss permanently.

So how do we do that? Intermittent fasting!

Chapter 5

What is intermittent fasting, and why should we do it?

There are only two states your body can be in at one time: fed or fasted. In fact, you are in one of those states right now! Even if you are a typical American who eats breakfast, lunch, and dinner (with snacks in between, because we have been told that the more meals we eat, the faster our metabolisms will run), you wake up each morning in a fasted state. The first meal of the day is called break-fast, because it's then that you break the nightly fast. So—congratulations! You are already fasting EVERY SINGLE DAY OF YOUR LIFE. Fasting doesn't sound quite so odd when you think of it that way, does it? You're already a faster, and you didn't know it!

So, now that we have determined that you ALREADY fast every single day, it's just a matter of extending the fast (unless you wake up at night to eat every few hours, in which case you are eating like a newborn...who specifically eats that way to gain body size...think about it). I'm pretty sure you don't wake up at night to eat, so we have confirmed that your body already knows how to fast.

But WHY should we fast? Ahh, that is the best part. Fasting gives us a metabolic advantage that other weight loss programs are missing.

Remember from the "calories" chapter—when our bodies perceive that we are in a caloric deficit, our

26

metabolisms slow to protect us. We saw that in the Biggest Loser study. The key to making any weight loss plan work for us is in keeping our bodies from perceiving that we are in a caloric deficit. That is where the magic of fasting comes in.

When your body becomes adapted to fasting (and you don't spike insulin during the fast; more about how to do that in the *Keeping the fast* chapter), you become a fat burning machine during the fast. Your body finally taps into your fat stores, and the energy you have stored on your body can power you throughout the day. That is what it is stored there for, after all!

Here is how the magic happens: because you have PLENTY of stored energy right there on your body, AND you can finally access it efficiently, your body does not get the signal that you are in an energy deficit. This is BIG NEWS, people! Your metabolism does not slow, as the Biggest Losers' metabolisms slowed.

Here is a link to a study that illustrates this phenomenon:

https://www.ncbi.nlm.nih.gov/pubmed/10837292

This study is called "Resting Energy Expenditure in Short-Term Starvation is Increased as a Result of an Increase in Serum Norepinephrine." That's a mouthful, but it's pretty exciting when you understand what "resting energy expenditure" means. So what is "resting energy expenditure"? It's how much energy your body burns while at rest. Don't let the word "starvation" scare you, though. When you are fasting, you aren't in danger of starvation. With an intermittent fasting schedule, you are only fasting "intermittently." It's in the name of it, after all.

In the conclusion of that study, the authors state, "Resting energy expenditure increases in early starvation, accompanied by an increase in plasma norepinephrine. This increase in norepinephrine seems to be due to a decline in serum glucose and may be the initial signal for metabolic changes in early starvation." Because of the fasting, resting energy expenditure went up, rather than down.

Besides increasing resting energy expenditure, intermittent fasting has other health benefits, which are being explored by the medical research community. Here is a link to a summary of some of the research:

https://www.ncbi.nlm.nih.gov/pmc/articles/PMC3946160/

The title of this article is called "Fasting: Molecular Mechanisms and Clinical Applications." I highly recommend that you read this article for yourself. It was released in 2014, and summarizes some of the benefits of various fasting protocols. It's exciting stuff. From the article: "As detailed in the remainder of this article, findings from well-controlled investigations in experimental animals, and emerging findings from human studies, indicate that different forms of fasting may provide effective strategies to reduce weight, delay aging, and optimize health." The authors go on to provide specific benefits from various research studies. The research they summarize has shown that fasting increases cognitive function, is anti-aging, may protect against cancer and various neurological diseases, and reduces inflammation.

Yes, this is an exciting time for research related to intermittent fasting! In fact, the 2016 Nobel Prize in Medicine was awarded to Yoshinori Ohsumi for his research related to a process called "autophagy." Here is a link to a summary of his research:

https://www.nobelprize.org/nobel_prizes/medicine/laureates/2016/press.html

What is autophagy? It is a process that occurs naturally within your own body. It's how your body breaks down excess cellular "junk." As an oversimplification, think of it as your body's own recycling system, and it's how your cells take out the garbage. Why do we need autophagy to happen? Over-accumulation of cellular "garbage" is responsible for various diseases or conditions related to aging. If you don't give your body a chance to clean out the garbage, it gunks up the whole system. Think about how this would look in your own household. If you stopped taking out the garbage, things would get out of control very quickly. Our bodies rely on the process of autophagy to maintain our healthy state. From the linked website, above: "Disrupted autophagy has been linked to Parkinson's disease, type 2 diabetes and other disorders that appear in the elderly. Mutations in autophagy genes can cause genetic disease. Disturbances in the autophagic machinery have also been linked to cancer." Whoa! As you can see, taking out the "cellular garbage" is pretty important!

What stimulates autophagy? If you guessed FASTING, then you are correct!

Autophagy has one other exciting benefit for those of us who are losing weight through intermittent fasting. Remember—during autophagy, your body is taking out the cellular garbage. As we lose weight through fasting, our bodies "eat up" the excess proteins hanging around in various places, and that can include excess skin. When people lose fat following a traditional low-calorie diet plan (where they don't get the benefits of autophagy), they can be left with saggy skin. You may have seen photos of people who have experienced extreme weight loss, and they are often left with so much excess skin that they need to have surgery to correct the problem. Dr. Fung (author of *The Obesity Code* and the *Intensive Dietary Management* blog) has worked with many patients in his medical practice, and he uses intermittent fasting to help them lose tremendous amounts of weight. He reports that his patients, who experience autophagy (thanks to fasting), don't have the problem of excess skin, even after losing in excess of 100 pounds. How exciting is that?

So—in this chapter, we have learned that we already fast every day, short-term fasting has been shown to rev up our metabolisms, and research on fasting shows many amazing health benefits. Instead of worrying that fasting is extreme or dangerous, we see that it's incredibly beneficial and on the cutting-edge of medical research.

Now that you know WHY you should fast, it's time to learn HOW!

NOTE: Since fasting has so many health benefits, you may be wondering if there is anyone who should not adopt a fasting lifestyle.

It's important to know that fasting is NOT appropriate for children or pregnant women.

Fasting is also not appropriate for anyone who has been diagnosed with an eating disorder. One important distinction between fasting and an eating disorder: fasting will not CAUSE you to develop an eating disorder, which is a psychological condition; but, if you suffer from an eating disorder, fasting can exacerbate it.

In addition, if you have any health conditions, you should consult a medical professional before beginning a fasting regimen.

And again—you should not take medical advice from me. You should always consult your doctor if you are in doubt.

Chapter 6

Finding your ideal intermittent fasting plan

There are many different intermittent fasting plans out there. I have included summaries of the books I have found to be most helpful in the annotated bibliography section of this book, and you can flip to that section to read about each one of them. Once you decide which intermittent fasting plan you want to try, I highly recommend that you research the plan for yourself by reading the original plan as written by its author. I have great respect for these authors, and each book on the list has shaped my thinking about intermittent fasting and why it is effective.

Personally, I have tried every type of intermittent fasting plan available. In fact, I started dabbling in intermittent fasting in about 2009. I never viewed it as a lifestyle, however, so I would try a plan briefly, and then fall off of the wagon. If you read my story in Appendix A, I have outlined it all there for you—the whole messy story. Instinctually I knew that intermittent fasting would be the answer for me as soon as I heard about it, but I never would commit or follow through, until I hit rock bottom in 2014. Once I realized that I no longer wanted to ride the weight-gain roller coaster, I was ready to commit. I finally understood that intermittent fasting was a lifestyle and not another diet plan, and I experimented until I found what works for me. The best part is that I have a whole toolbox full of intermittent fasting strategies that I can pull out when I need them, to suit my current situation. I can pick and choose which strategies to implement based on how I want to live my life.

In a nutshell, there are two main types of intermittent fasting strategies: plans you do every day (an "eating window" approach), or plans you implement a certain number of times per week (an "up/down day" approach).

Which approach to intermittent fasting is the best? It's the one that makes you feel in control and the one that you can follow long-term as a lifestyle. That's important to understand from the beginning—intermittent fasting is a lifestyle. It isn't something that you start today and then end when you get to some arbitrary "goal weight." Something you start and then stop is a DIET. Intermittent fasting isn't a diet—as I said, it's a lifestyle.

Before I get into the specifics of an eating window approach vs. an up/down day approach, I want to talk about hormones again. From the insulin chapter, you may recall that insulin is the key to fat storage vs. fat burning. If you keep insulin as low as possible in your body, you are able to burn fat. If insulin is high, your body wants to store fat. Insulin is the key hormone to understand if you want to lose weight and keep it off long-term.

Insulin isn't, however, the only hormone that affects your results. There are other hormonal regulators of appetite, as described in this paper, which is called, surprisingly, "Hormonal Regulators of Appetite":

https://www.ncbi.nlm.nih.gov/pmc/articles/PMC2777281/

This paper explains, in a very science-y way, how ghrelin and leptin work together to give you signals related to your food intake and how much fat you have stored on your body. To overly simplify a very complex process, ghrelin tells us that we need to eat, and leptin tells us that we have had enough. If your body is sensitive to both ghrelin and leptin, and everything is working as it should, you will

32

remain at your ideal weight effortlessly, and your appetite will tell you when to eat and when to stop. We are born with these hormones working perfectly in concert with one another. A baby doesn't know how many calories he has had, but he gets hunger signals to let him know that it is time to eat. If you have ever tried to feed a toddler who isn't hungry, you have seen that it can be impossible. If they aren't hungry, they aren't going to eat, which is how we should all live our lives. Children come to us with appetite hormones that are working perfectly, and then we force them to eat at mealtimes on an arbitrary schedule, and then we feed them highly processed foods, both of which work together to cause our kids to completely lose sight of their satiety signals. Thanks, mom.

When we follow restrictive diets, count calories, eat according to an arbitrary meal schedule, etc., we disconnect from our satiety hormones. We eat because it is time to eat. We eat because food is available. The more we do it, the worse shape we are in.

Bottom line, if you have had trouble sticking to a diet, it isn't your fault—it's your hormones. The overwhelming drive to eat is coming from ghrelin, telling you to eat more. You are no longer able to get the signals from leptin, telling you that you have had enough. Understand that uncontrollable or constant hunger is a sign that you have made some dietary choices that aren't working for you. On the other hand, satiety is a good sign, telling you that your body is happy with what you are doing.

So, why am I mentioning this here, in the chapter on finding your perfect intermittent fasting plan? Stick with me. If you flip to the back and read my description of Dr. Herring's second book, *AC: The Power of Appetite Correction*, in the annotated bibliography, you'll see my explanation of the state he calls "appetite correction," or AC. (You really should buy his book and read what he has to say; it's worth it!) What he calls "appetite correction" is actually a state of regulated hormones. You suddenly have leptin and ghrelin working as they should, and part of this is because you can access your fat stores appropriately due to low levels of circulating insulin. You eat according to appetite and never have to count another calorie again, because you have gotten your hormones back into the state that nature intended. Hallelujah, and pass the collection plate. (*You may not get that joke if you aren't a southerner...*)

Remember this when you are experimenting to find your ideal intermittent fasting plan: you need to look for the one that gives you this hormonal correction Dr. Herring describes as appetite correction. It won't happen overnight, as it takes time to undo years of damage. Once you get there, though, you'll know, because you'll have a level of peace around food that you have never had in recent memory. You can pass up cake, because you are full. When I stick to my preferred intermittent fasting lifestyle, I live in a state of balance, where ghrelin and leptin work together to control my appetite, just as nature intended.

In the next two chapters, I'll summarize both the eating window approach and the up/down day approach to help you decide which might be the best fit for your lifestyle.

Then, in the next chapter, I'll describe my own preferred approach to intermittent fasting, called the One Meal a Day (OMAD) lifestyle. Even if the name of it sounds overly restrictive, and you are hesitant to commit to such an "extreme" plan, I suggest that you read that chapter with an open mind. I have found my own best results and the most dietary freedom with the OMAD lifestyle. It's the plan that gets my hormones into balance the best. If you had told me that five years ago, I would have refused to believe it, but it is true.

Chapter 7

An "eating window" approach to intermittent fasting

In an eating window intermittent fasting plan, you set a specific period of time for your daily eating "window," and all caloric food/beverages must be consumed within that period of time. As soon as the first bite of food/sip of caloric beverage enters your mouth, your window is "open," and when you take your last bite/sip, it is "closed." I have seen eating windows as short as one hour and windows as long as 10-12 hours. I would never personally consider or even recommend a 10-12 hour eating window; that's just not enough fasting for most people to get the results they are hoping for. An eating window somewhere between 1-8 hours is more typical and should give most people better results.

My first foray into an eating window was the Fast 5 plan, written by Dr. Bert Herring. In Dr. Herring's plan, you have a daily 5-hour eating window. I think that a 5-hour window is a great starting point for many people, but you will need to experiment with a variety of window lengths to find what works for you.

While personally experimenting with window-length, I also tried an 8-hour eating window, which is one promoted by other intermittent fasters. For me, 8 hours is just too long, and I don't lose any weight following an 8-hour eating window. That doesn't mean that an 8-hour window won't be perfect for YOU; it just doesn't work at all for ME. As I said, you should experiment to find which window length works best for you. Our bodies are all very different, and what works for me might not be the best plan for you.

In the Fast 5 plan, which I suggest as a great starting point, Dr. Herring personally uses the 5 p.m.-10 p.m. period of time for his window. He does say that you can choose whatever 5-hour window works best for you, but I think his recommendation for 5-10 p.m. is genius. Let me explain. When I first started, I wanted to maximize the number of eating opportunities available to me, so I used a 12:30-5:30 eating window. That allowed me to eat a full lunch and a full dinner every day. Sounds great, doesn't it? Well, if you are like me, you can fit a lot of food into a full lunch and a full dinner. Weight loss was VERY slow because I was eating a LOT of food every day.

When I re-read Dr. Herring's book, I realized that several times throughout it, he mentioned eating "one meal" each day in your 5-hour window, and suddenly everything clicked into place for me. Instead of trying to maximize eating opportunities, I needed to find a window that would allow me to feel satisfied, but without two full meals every day. When I shifted my window to one that opened at 5 p.m., I had much better results. The timing of my 5-hour eating window made a tremendous difference in my overall success.

I don't always wait until 5 p.m. every single day to open my window, but I do aim for one real meal each day within a window that is no more than 5 hours. This is what I usually do, but I'm not psycho about it. I want this to be a lifestyle that I adjust to suit me, rather than something that controls my life in a rigid manner. It's fine to open my window with a snack, and eat a meal later; or, I might choose to open my window with a meal and then eat a snack later. Some days, I eat one meal only, and that's it. I listen to my body, and on days that I am hungrier, I eat more. On days when I am not as hungry, I eat less. I don't calculate

36

calories, and I don't restrict any foods—though I do pay attention to how certain foods make me feel.

Now that I pay more attention to satiety signals (thanks, appetite and satiety hormones), my thoughts are no longer about how much food I can cram into a 5-hour window, which has made it work much better for me. I don't even really track my window anymore—but when I do, I find that a 2-3 hour window is enough for most days. If you had told me five years ago that I would be happily eating one real meal per day, and limiting all intake to a 2-3 hour window most days, I would have run screaming from the idea. It sounds crazily restrictive! In actuality, I have never had the peace around food that I have now. I genuinely eat whatever I want every day until I am full and satisfied. It feels too good to be true, but it IS true.

One of the benefits of an intermittent fasting plan with a daily eating window is that it is easy to fall into a rhythm. Your body learns to expect food at a certain time each day, and once you adjust to that schedule, it becomes easy. In fact, I find it to be easier than eating all day long. You don't have to make any food decisions until your window opens. No constant thoughts of "should I eat this now?" because when the window is closed, it's closed. I used to have many thoughts about eating during a typical day, and now I don't. It is so much more peaceful. If you have never fasted before, that might sound unbelievable, but once you get used to it, it is such a great way to live.

Notice that I mentioned in the previous paragraph how easy it is "once you adjust." I'm going to be honest with you here—the adjustment period can be the hardest part of implementing an intermittent fasting regimen, and it is why many people fail. When you first start, your body is used to being in a fed-state during the day. This means that your body is used to running off of your circulating blood glucose and stored glycogen for energy. As soon as you run out of ready energy, your body sends a signal for you to eat, and you fuel back up with a snack, a meal, or that afternoon latte. When you begin fasting, however, you don't give in to those signals to eat, and your body can get MAD at you. The signals to eat keep coming. You might feel shaky, tired, or get a headache. You may even feel a little sick to your stomach. These feelings can be unpleasant, and if you eat, you'll feel better immediately. It's the number one reason most people give me for being unwilling to try intermittent fasting: they "can't," because they get headaches and "low blood sugar." This adjustment period is a barrier for many—but I want to encourage you to commit to a week or two before you decide that you "can't" fast.

Here's the thing you need to remember: your goal is to start burning your own fat for fuel. The ONLY WAY to tap into that stored fat is to STOP running on glucose/glycogen. You can either be a fat-burner or a sugar-burner. The end. Making the transition from a sugar-burner to a fat-burner is the hard part, but once you do it, you will be AMAZED at how good you feel. I promise.

Take today. I'm writing this at 4:45 p.m. I'm starting to get some mild hunger signals because my body anticipates that I will break my fast within the next hour or two. (No, I don't start shoving food into my mouth as soon as 5:00 hits…anymore…though there have been days like that.) Today I wrote for several hours, then went to visit some friends. I jumped on the trampoline with their children. While there, I refused to eat some jellybeans that I was offered (apparently, they might be delicious, or they might be "booger" flavored…you can't tell from looking at them…it's some sort of fun surprise in every bite…thank goodness that fasting saved me from that fate). I ran a few errands and then came back home to more writing. I haven't felt tired or lethargic for one moment all day. Contrast that with yesterday—which just happened to be Christmas Day. Because intermittent fasting is flexible, I opened my window at noon with a Christmas brunch. I was ready for a nap by 2 p.m., and I needed a cup of coffee mid-afternoon to keep me going. Then I had to have a snack before dinner. Then dinner. Oof. I thoroughly enjoyed my time with family, but I didn't enjoy the way I felt after eating all of that food.

The lesson that I want to share is this: I feel better today, fasting, than I did yesterday when I began eating at noon. I didn't have MORE energy from my frequent meals, and actually, I had profoundly LESS energy. This is because it takes a surprising amount of energy to digest food, and I notice that whenever I open my window early in the day, I get a distinct afternoon slump. When I'm fasting, I don't get that slump. Ever. (In fact, one reason I gave up alternate day fasting, which I discuss in the next chapter, is that when I do a full fast over 24 hours in length, I can't sleep at night— I have so much energy that it keeps me awake.)

When you first start fasting, you will be stuck in that in-between transition period that I already mentioned. Your body will yell at you to EAT, because it's used to running on glucose/glycogen. You are going to be grumpy. Tired. HANGRY. Trust me—the promised-land is around the corner, once you make that transition to fat burning. Once you get past the transition, you'll wonder how you ever managed to eat all day long.

There are several ways to make the transition easier. One idea is to gradually shorten your eating window until you find a length that works for you. Start with skipping breakfast. Gradually push back your lunchtime every day, until you are breaking your fast in the late afternoon. This is a sensible approach that many people use when beginning an intermittent fasting lifestyle.

Another way to make the transition easier involves a temporary change in WHAT you are eating during the day. (Notice that I said it is temporary—I don't restrict anything in my diet, and I am not going to ask you to do it, either.) Years ago, in the 90s, I read a diet book called *The Carbohydrate Addict's Diet*. In this plan, you eat a low carb breakfast, a low carb lunch, and then for dinner, you have a "reward meal" of whatever you want. You must eat that reward meal in a time period that is one hour or shorter. (In hindsight, I realize that the authors developed a type of intermittent fasting plan, well before the phrase "intermittent fasting" had been coined.)

So, why is a temporary shift to a low carb eating plan for two of your meals helpful? If you think back to the chapter on insulin and weight loss, you remember that when you have a lot of insulin circulating in your system, you won't burn fat. Fasting lowers insulin, but low carb diets also lower insulin (not as much as fasting, but enough to help you get started). If you make sure that your low carb breakfast and lunch are "low carb/high fat," also known as LCHF or Ketogenic-style ("Keto") eating, it helps your body get into a fat burning state. (Tip: search the internet for some suggestions of what to eat for your LCHF/Ketogenic meals. I could not eat that way forever, but remember—I am not asking you to, either.)

You can use this strategy to smooth your transition to an intermittent fasting eating window. Begin by having a LCHF breakfast and a LCHF lunch, plus a dinner of whatever you want, that you finish within a one-hour period to limit the length of time that you are releasing insulin (it ALWAYS comes back to insulin). Soon you should be able to skip breakfast, and then eventually you'll be able to painlessly skip lunch. Voila! You are an intermittent faster! You'll also find that it's easier to skip breakfast and lunch than it is to prepare two LCHF meals. Intermittent fasting…the diet for people too lazy to cook a bunch of meals during the day!

I was never able to lose weight following *The Carbohydrate Addict's Diet*, but temporarily eating LCHF during the day can really help your body through the adjustment period. Don't expect fast weight loss, but instead think of it as a stepping-stone to reaching your intermittent fasting window, as you become a fat-burner rather than a sugar-burner. (Funny side note: the author of *The Carbohydrate Addict's Diet*, Dr. Rachael Heller, actually lost a great deal of weight and kept it off long-term, but she wasn't following the plan in the diet book she released. When you read her story, you see that what she did was skip breakfast and lunch every day, and then she ate dinner only. It worked like a charm for her. Remember though; this book was released during the 90s. "Fasting" was not something that people were considering for weight loss. Even though Dr. Heller lost her weight by eating one meal per day, she developed a plan that had you eating the more typical pattern of breakfast, lunch, and dinner. I assume it was because she felt that it would be an easier sell.)

What if the idea of a daily eating window sounds too restrictive for you? Good news—you may prefer an "up/down day" fasting strategy. The next chapter will explain how those plans work.

Chapter 8

An "up/down day" intermittent fasting approach

In an up/down day intermittent fasting approach, every day is either a regular eating ("up") day, or a fasting ("down") day. There are many patterns of fasting/eating days to choose from, and you can vary approaches to see what works for you.

In most of these up/down day approaches, you aren't required to do full fasts on your down days. Instead, you are allowed up to 500 calories on those days. These plans (as written by the original authors) aren't true fasts. You still reap many of the benefits of fasting, and the up/down pattern of eating works well to prevent the metabolic adaptation you find in a typical low-calorie diet (remember the Biggest Loser study, which you read about in the chapter about calories). Even though you are allowed to have 500 calories, think back to the lessons we have learned in the chapter on insulin. You don't want to have frequent insulin release on your fasting days, so structure your intake for maximum fat burning potential. See the chapter on what you can have while fasting for specific tips to avoid insulin release during the fasting period.

While these plans "allow" you to have up to 500 calories on the down days, I prefer to reap as many benefits from the fasting period as possible. For that reason, when I have a down day, I do an actual fast with 0 calories (other than the negligible calorie content from black coffee). I have found that, for me, it is easier to abstain from food completely for 36 hours than it is to limit myself to 500 calories. You are free to experiment to see what works best for you—the way that is "best" is the one that you will stick to with the least amount of discomfort on fasting days.

The way I work a down day is this: I wake up, and stick to black coffee/water/sparkling water all day, until bedtime. I go to bed without having eaten anything all day. The next day when I wake up, it's an up day, and I am free to break the fast whenever I want. If I break the fast with breakfast, I have fasted for approximately 36 hours. If I wait until lunch to break the fast, I have fasted for about 42 hours.

There are several specific plans that you can choose from if considering an up/down day approach to intermittent fasting. The most extreme version of up/down day fasting is called "Alternate Day Fasting," or ADF. ADF is exactly how it sounds: one day you fast, and the next day you eat according to whatever schedule you want. It continues indefinitely in the alternate day pattern. ADF is heavily researched by Dr. Krista Varady, and she explains her findings in the book *The Every Other Day Diet*. *The Alternate-Day Diet*, by Dr. Johnson, is another book that recommends an alternate day approach. Both Dr. Varady and Dr. Johnson recommend that you count calories on your fasting days. Dr. Johnson also suggests calorie counting on your regular eating days. Dr. Varady claims that according to her research, people rarely overdo it on the up days, and weight loss occurs at a consistent pace without calorie counting. You can decide which approach appeals to you most. Personally, I don't want to count calories, EVER. Maybe that is one additional reason that I choose to do a full fast on my version of the down days: it's easy to count to 0.

At the other end of the up/down day spectrum is a plan generally referred to as 5:2. The numbers 5 and 2 stand for the number of days of the week that you do it. The first number is how many regular eating days you have per week (5), and the second number is how many fasting days you have per week (2). In 5:2, you can choose any 2 days to have as your fasting days, and you eat "normally" for the other 5 days of the week. Remember—just like with ADF, you are allowed to have up to 500 calories on the fasting days, though I always stick to 0 calories.

5:2 is a great plan for many reasons, and one of the main attractions is the fact that you are only restricting the foods you eat for 2 days per week, and the rest of the time you eat normally. For me, one of the main drawbacks to 5:2 is also the fact that you are only restricting the foods you eat for 2 days per week, and the rest of the time you eat normally. 5 days of eating normally per week is just too much food for me. I don't lose weight on 5:2, but it is a great maintenance plan for me. I maintained my weight throughout the summer of 2015 by following 5:2 from April – August. For specifics on how to use 5:2, you can read more about the plan in *The 5:2 Diet*, by Kate Harrison or *The Fast Diet*, by Michael Mosley and Mimi Spencer.

If ADF sounds like too much fasting, and 5:2 doesn't sound like enough, I suggest you try a plan called 4:3. As with 5:2, the first number stands for the number of days where you eat normally (4), and the second number stands for the number of fasting days each week (3). I lose weight (though slowly) when following 4:3, so it works better for me as a weight loss plan than 5:2, which strictly works for me as a maintenance plan.

When you use ADF, 4:3, or 5:2, you need to consider how you want to schedule your week. One problem I always had with true ADF was timing. There are 7 days per week, and so that means that one week you fast on Monday, Wednesday, Friday, and Sunday, and the next week you fast on Tuesday, Thursday, and Saturday. I don't want to do a full fast on a Friday or a Saturday—ever—and I prefer to have more of a predictable routine to my fasting. Therefore, for weight loss, rather than true ADF, I would use a 4:3 routine that looked like this: I would fast on Sunday, Tuesday, and Thursday, leaving me with Friday and

Saturday as up days for weekend social events. If I had an event scheduled for Sunday, Tuesday, or Thursday, I would either fast through it or rearrange my fasting schedule to suit. (Fasting through an event is always an option. Nobody really notices whether you eat or not—plus, I have found that I am less willing to eat something just because it is there, and the food has to be worth it.) When I used 5:2 for maintenance, I would fast on Monday and Thursday each week. I was always ready for a good fast on Monday after the weekend, and then Thursday I fasted in preparation for the upcoming weekend. This routine worked very well for me. As with 4:3, I could always rearrange my fasting days if I had a special event.

Up/down day intermittent fasting plans such as ADF, 5:2, and 4:3 are very popular, because many people really like the idea of having some days where you don't have to think about "dieting," and you can eat like everyone else. That was one of the attractions for me, as well. I found that over time, however, I had some problems with both 5:2 and 4:3. I started to dread the fasting days, and one reason for that is that I don't sleep well after fasting all day. I also didn't enjoy the up days nearly as much as I thought I would. I spent all day thinking about what I should eat next, or deciding if it was time to eat, or calculating how much time until I could eat. I had SO MANY THOUGHTS ABOUT FOOD that it wore me out. Plus, I fell victim to the afternoon slump on the eating days. I'm not saying I will never use ADF, 5:2, or 4:3 again, but for now, I prefer the one meal a day (OMAD) approach, which I will describe in the next chapter.

Chapter 9

One meal a day: My sweet spot

As I already mentioned in the chapter on using an eating window approach to intermittent fasting, I started my intermittent fasting journey by using Dr. Bert Herring's plan called Fast 5. When I first started, I arranged my 5-hour daily eating window so I could maximize the number of eating opportunities in the day. I was fasting for 19 hours each day, but I was eating two full meals during my window. Of course, weight loss was s-l-o-w.

Weight loss was so slow, in fact, that I experimented with some extreme calorie restriction within my 5-hour window. You can read about that in my full weight loss story, which is in Appendix A. The extreme calorie restriction did speed up my rate of loss, but I was miserable. This was also before I read any of Dr. Fung's work on the dangers of prolonged calorie restriction, and before the Biggest Loser study was released. Thankfully, I didn't have the discipline to either count or restrict calories for long, so I didn't do any long-term metabolic damage that I have been able to detect. I do not recommend that you follow my example: NO extreme calorie restriction for you!

At that point, I re-read the Fast 5 book, and suddenly something jumped out at me. Dr. Herring said, more than once, that during your 5-hour window, "you're only eating one meal a day." That is a direct quote from his FAQ chapter, in fact. No wonder weight loss was so slow when I crammed in two meals! In late January of 2015, I started officially eating one meal a day with no conscious calorie restriction, and effortlessly reached my goal weight of 135 pounds by mid-March. (I have gone on to lose a few more pounds since then. How many? I don't know. I no longer weigh myself. See the chapter on weighing to find out why!)

After reaching my goal weight, I still wasn't convinced that I wanted to fast every day. Eating one meal a day worked, but did I really want to eat like that for the rest of my life? At that point, I switched over to 5:2 for maintenance. I used 5:2 from May-August to maintain my weight. I did full fasts of at least 36 hours for 2 days per week, and I ate normally for the other 5 days. It worked like a charm.

As you know, I am a teacher, so I was on summer break from the end of May-early August. When school started back in August, I continued using 5:2; however, I suddenly had a problem. I had to pack a lunch on my up days! I realized that I didn't WANT to pack a lunch. Ever. I also didn't feel like eating breakfast before school. It became crystal clear: I am TOO LAZY for 5:2. (Not really, but— okay—that is part of it. I don't want to have to think about breakfast or lunch when I'm working. You can call me lazy if you want. I don't mind.)

At that point, I thought back to my epiphany from March about eating one meal a day, and decided that was going to be my plan going forward. I started a "one meal a day" Facebook group on August 24, 2015, with just me and my husband as members. (He doesn't do intermittent fasting—but I learned that you can't start a group with just yourself, so I needed him in there to keep me company.) Eventually, I recruited some of my other intermittent fasting friends, and we began to form a community of people who realized that there is a great deal of freedom to be found in a one meal a day (OMAD) lifestyle. As of December 2016, we reached 3,500 members in our group, and the number is still climbing. Many of the testimonials in Appendix D are from members of the OMAD Facebook group. It's the friendliest Facebook group I have ever been in, and the members are extremely supportive of one another. I guess that is because we have found a lifestyle that just WORKS! No need to be grumpy or hangry when you have such a great weight loss/maintenance plan!

Besides being a convenient plan for someone who doesn't want to pack a lunch, like me, some research indicates that eating one meal a day has a metabolic advantage when compared to eating all meals spread out throughout the day.

https://www.ncbi.nlm.nih.gov/pubmed/17413096

The study from that link is called "A Controlled Trial of Reduced Meal Frequency Without Caloric Restriction in Healthy, Normal-weight, Middle-aged Adults." The researchers found that subjects eating only one meal a day lost significantly more fat than those eating the same exact number of calories in a more-typical three meals per day pattern. (Sorry, CI/CO, you lose AGAIN!) If you think back to the two chapters on calories and insulin, this is just what we would expect to see happen. When you are fasting during the day, and keeping insulin low, you unlock your fat stores. The body learns to burn fat preferentially for energy, and you become a fat burning machine! Your body revs up your metabolism in response to the fast. In contrast, when you try to eat frequently throughout the day, your body doesn't dip into your fat stores as readily due to the frequent release of insulin. If you are in any type of energy deficit, your body may burn muscle instead of fat (because your fat stores are locked away—thanks, insulin!)

When fasting all day, you burn fat preferentially. Amazing! Then, you are able to eat a delicious meal of whatever you want for dinner. Even if you eat 1,500-2,000 calories in your one meal, you'll likely be in a caloric deficit. No, I am not suggesting that you count calories, because I still believe that the practice of calorie counting is flawed and tedious. I eat until I am satisfied, and I stop when I am full. It is truly liberating. I only mention it because it seems incredible that you can eat that much food in a meal and not GAIN weight.

Here's the thing, though. I am pretty sure that I do not eat as many calories in my one meal as I would have eaten if I spread out my meals over the course of the day. I am certain that I eat less when I follow a one meal a day lifestyle. I have learned to listen to my satiety signals, and I stop when I have had enough. I don't need to count calories or even worry about food intake. Some days, I am hungrier, so I eat more. Some days, I get full really fast, so I eat less. I don't worry about eating too much OR not eating enough, because when the body's hormones are working properly, we naturally adjust intake to meet our body's needs. Think about it—animals in the wild don't count calories, and they are not obese. It's only when we put animals on a feeding schedule that they develop weight problems. (Think about all of the overweight pets, and compare them to animals in the wild, who effortlessly maintain their ideal weight.)

One caveat--don't expect your satiety signals to be perfectly in tune at first. It takes a while for your body to learn to listen to your hormones again. You may even find that you tend to binge-eat for the first week or two. Dr. Herring addresses this in his *Fast 5* book and calls it "compensatory over-eating." Some people even GAIN weight at first, due to initial overeating. Yikes! Nothing makes a plan seem more terrible than sticking to it faithfully and actually GAINING weight. Here's the thing, though. Once you spend a few weeks following an intermittent fasting lifestyle, your hormones get back into balance, and you once again become in tune with your satiety signals. You don't need to count calories, just like the lean animals in the wild don't have to count calories.

I haven't been specific about how long your window should be for you to be officially living the OMAD lifestyle.

I did that purposefully. I am not going to tell you what your window length has to be. So there.

If you eat one meal a day, and fast according to the recommendations in this book for a large portion of your day, you are living the OMAD lifestyle. If you snack all day until dinner and only eat dinner, you are NOT living the OMAD lifestyle. If you drink diet soda all day until dinner and then eat dinner only, you are also NOT following the OMAD lifestyle. You are on a calorie-restricted diet, because you are constantly spiking your insulin. See the chapter on what you should consume during the fast for a specific list of what is or is not allowed. If you aren't following those recommendations, you are not fasting effectively, and I don't want to hear about it when you experience a plateau or weight regain.

The key to the OMAD lifestyle is that you are following the guidelines for fasting most of the day, and you are eating only one real meal most days. That doesn't mean that you have to limit yourself to one plate of food or eat within a one-hour window. The last thing I want to do is shovel in food so I can meet some arbitrary deadline. Once again, that is diet mentality, and not a pleasant lifestyle. I no longer time my eating window most days, and it is an incredibly freeing way to live.

Let's see how this could look. What if I drink black coffee and water until 4 p.m., and then I eat a snack at 4. I eat dinner at 7 p.m., and then I eat dessert at 8 p.m., at which time I close my eating window because I am satisfied. Did I follow a one meal a day lifestyle? I hope you said yes, because that is a perfect example of the flexibility you have when following OMAD. It was one real meal, plus a snack, plus dessert, all within a 4 hour time period.

On another day I might eat dinner at 6 p.m., and by 6:30 I am full and satisfied. Is that OMAD? Why, yes, it is! Am I practicing calorie restriction? NO, because I am full and satisfied. My hormones told me I had enough that day.

For me, the OMAD intermittent fasting lifestyle is incredibly flexible. I have learned to listen to my body, and on days where I am hungrier, I will have a longer eating window. On days when I am less hungry, I eat a smaller meal. It feels like a lifestyle rather than a diet, because I am not controlled by a bunch of rules. If I have a special occasion that includes brunch, I will eat more than one meal that day, and it's okay—because, in a lifestyle, every day doesn't have to be perfect (because this isn't a religion).

Are you ready for a trick question? What about this: if I eat brunch at 11:00 a.m., and then dinner at 6:00 p.m., did I follow OMAD? The answer is NO. Remember, though—it is okay to deviate for a special occasion every now and then. I didn't cheat—I had a planned indulgence. I don't do that often, so it is fine. I am still living the OMAD lifestyle. It isn't a jail sentence; it's a lifestyle.

If you are following the OMAD lifestyle to lose weight, you probably don't want to be quite as flexible with your window length or planned indulgences as I am in maintenance. When I was in weight loss mode, I did generally stick to an eating window of about an hour many days. I also didn't include dessert as often. Intermittent fasting has many advantages over regular diets, but it isn't magic. It is possible to have such a luxurious window that you will stop losing weight, or even gain weight. This is where you have to be honest with yourself. You can't have seven snacks, dessert, and one huge meal and expect great results. Sorry.

The good news is that when I follow the OMAD lifestyle consistently, fasting properly during the day, and eating only one real meal each evening, my satiety signals are pretty strong, and I don't overeat often. Last night I didn't eat dessert, because I didn't want it! I was literally too full to eat cake!

As I already mentioned, Dr. Herring (of Fast 5) wrote a second book that I highly recommend, and it is called *AC: The Power of Appetite Correction*. Appetite correction (AC) is the Holy Grail of intermittent fasting, and it is the state you reach when your satiety signals are in tune with an appropriate amount of food for your body. The OMAD lifestyle gives me fantastic AC, which is why it is so easy for me to follow. I highly encourage you to experiment with various window lengths or fasting approaches until you find AC.

Chapter 10

Keeping the fast: What can I have when I'm fasting?

This may be the most important chapter in the whole book, because you absolutely can fast incorrectly and sabotage your results. If you don't keep the fast properly, you will not see the type of long-term results that you are looking for (even if you get great short-term results). Your goal may be to lose weight, but fast weight loss isn't the only measure of success when you are intermittent fasting. If your only goal is to lose weight fast, I can give you several recommendations for that. Of course, you'll be sorry in the long run. Reread the Biggest Loser study section and think about whether you want to live your life in a constant state of deprivation. I sure don't.   No, our goal isn't fast weight loss. Balancing our hormones (insulin, ghrelin, and leptin) so they work the way they are supposed to—that is our goal. Once you do that, weight loss will follow, and eventually, it will feel effortless. Take care of your body, and it will take care of you.

First of all, remember this—as I explained in a previous chapter, there's so much more to weight loss than calories in/calories out (CI/CO), and most intermittent fasting plans do not require calorie counting in any way, shape, or form during your eating window or on an up day. Even so, you want to stick to zero calories during the fast for best results (because if you are eating or ingesting calories in any form, you clearly aren't fasting). Even more importantly, you want to keep your insulin from spiking.

That's the only way you are going to access your stored fat for fuel—and face it—that is why we are fasting to begin with. Burn, baby, burn!

So what causes insulin to spike? Well, foods do, but we already know that we shouldn't be eating if we are fasting. The really sneaky thing that you need to understand is that even zero-calorie beverages and "diet" products can cause your insulin to spike. You could be ingesting zero calories during your fasting period and STILL be spiking your insulin constantly. If that happens, you are not going to be able to access your stored fat very well. Your body won't burn fat during the fast, and you will miss out on the metabolism-boosting effects of a true fast. Because your body doesn't have access to your stored fat for energy, your body is going to perceive that you are in an energy deficit. What does your body do when you are in a prolonged energy deficit? It SLOWS your metabolism, as we saw in the Biggest Loser study.

Just to recap for emphasis: by spiking insulin during the day, you will not access your stored fat effectively, and you risk slowing your metabolism. When you understand that, you realize that the last thing you would ever want to do is spike insulin by ingesting the wrong thing during the fast.

So what DOES cause insulin to spike, other than food or calories? It's sweetness. When we taste something sweet, our bodies "know" that calories are entering the body and insulin is released to deal with the expected rise in blood sugar. The only problem is that in the modern era, we have figured out how to make things that taste sweet and don't actually have any calories. We have created artificial sweeteners and artificial flavors in the lab that have all of the sweetness but none of the calories. We think we are making a good choice, because we "know" that it's calories that make us gain weight. Anything with zero calories seems perfect for the dieter. Except the opposite is true. You are sabotaging your success, and you don't even know it.

54

If you search for information about various sweeteners and insulin release, you'll find all sorts of contradictory information. Many websites (and studies) seem to suggest that certain sweeteners are safe, and other websites or studies say the opposite. It can be really hard to know who is right.

Here is a link that might help. It takes you to the abstract of a study about sweet tastes and insulin release. Insulin release is referred to here as "CPIR," for "cephalic phase insulin release."

https://www.ncbi.nlm.nih.gov/m/pubmed/17510492/

This is what they found: "From these results, we conclude that sweetness information conducted by this taste nerve provides essential information for eliciting CPIR." Pay attention to that. They found that sweetness caused "CPIR," which is insulin release. Even before blood glucose went up, insulin had already been released—from just the sweet taste!

Here's something else from the study that is quite interesting. When they cut the nerve from the taste receptors, no insulin was released in response to the sweet flavors. This is HUGE to help us understand the insulin response of sweet tastes. When the sweet flavors were no longer detectable by the brain, insulin was not released. This clearly illustrates that the perception of the sweet taste by the brain is essential. In everyday language: if you taste sweetness, you release insulin.

Here's another study related to insulin release and sweet tastes:

https://www.ncbi.nlm.nih.gov/m/pubmed/18556090/

In this second study, the participants didn't even ingest the sweetened liquid fully—they merely swished it around in their mouths and spat it out. From the abstract: "A significant increase of plasma insulin concentration was apparent after stimulation with sucrose and saccharin. In conclusion, the current data suggest that the sweeteners sucrose and saccharin activate a CPIR even when applied to the oral cavity only."

The subjects in that experiment swished around sweet liquids and then spat them out. Even though they didn't ingest anything, their insulin was raised in responses to the sweet taste. (*Note: some people get nervous at this point and start to worry about brushing their teeth or using mouthwash. Think about it this way. Yes, you may have a sweet taste in your mouth BRIEFLY from brushing your teeth or using mouthwash, but the duration isn't going to be for long. Everyone who knows you has asked me to tell you—please don't stop brushing your teeth or using mouthwash. As long as you don't use it every hour on the hour, you should be fine. Your family and friends thank you.*)

So—what's the takeaway from these two studies on sweet tastes and insulin release? When you read somewhere on the internet that aspartame doesn't cause insulin release, or stevia doesn't cause insulin release, or _____ does not cause insulin release, etc., remember these studies. A sweet taste=insulin release, even in the absence of calories.

If you are drinking artificially sweetened and/or sweet/fruity flavored beverages during your fast, now you should understand that you are going to constantly spike your insulin levels. With raised insulin levels, you won't access your stored fat as readily, and your body may burn muscle mass rather than fat. Remember—a lot of circulating insulin prevents fat burning. When you aren't burning fat for fuel, you will end up with a slowed metabolism rather than a faster metabolism, AND you may end up with less muscle mass. It may sound like I am repeating myself with this message, and...GOOD! I am. I keep repeating myself because I want you to understand this very important piece of the puzzle. In order for you to find lasting success, you have to lower your insulin levels so you can burn fat during the fast.

I had a REALLY hard time with this, personally, because I did NOT want to drink my coffee black. I used vanilla flavored stevia, and it made me happy to have that sweet flavor in my coffee. I drank a LOT of coffee with stevia during my fasting time, in fact. I thought it wasn't affecting me, because I was losing weight. I also drank sweet fruity teas with names like "baked apple." Eventually, I struggled with a little bit of weight regain, and told myself that it was normal to regain a little weight. I had to work to get about 8 pounds off that I had previously lost. That's normal, right? Maintenance is hard. That's what we have been told, after all.

Then, I read Dr. Fung's book, *The Obesity Code*, and finally understood what I was risking by spiking my insulin during the fast. I pitched a fit (that's what we do here in the South), I whined, and I moaned…and I gave up stevia. I started drinking my coffee black. And…I didn't die. In a week or two, I was fully used to the taste of black coffee.

The better news is that I was able to lose the 8 pounds of weight regain, and I have slowly continued to lose fat here and there with zero effort, ever since. Eliminating the stevia (and the fruity and sweet tasting teas) made a huge difference in my results, and I am confident that I won't have trouble with regain in the future. (In fact, my waist got smaller this year from November 14th – December 14th, which means I lost some fat over Thanksgiving. How many people lose weight over the holidays?) More importantly, ditching the stevia has made an enormous difference in my level of appetite correction. It is much easier for me to fast during the day now, and I am more in tune with my satiety signals than ever before. Lowering insulin levels during my fast by eliminating stevia has made a huge difference for me. Stevia, you are dead to me.

So now we fully understand that we don't want to spike insulin during the fast. You may find yourself wondering what you CAN have. Please refer to the following lists to see what you should and shouldn't ingest during the fast.

Allowed during the fast in any quantity:
- **Water**
- **Black coffee** (*unflavored*)
- **Teas** (*unflavored green tea, black tea, etc., where the only ingredient is some variety of "tea" with no added flavors*)
- **Herbal teas** (*Select ones that are not fruity or sweet. Especially avoid the fruity and sweet ones that list "natural flavor" in the ingredient list*)
- **Sparkling water** like La Croix, Perrier, and San Pellegrino (*select the unflavored varieties, as the fruit flavors can spike insulin*)

Possibly okay to have small amounts during the adjustment phase only, but use SPARINGLY:
Note: It's important to know that I avoid everything on this list personally, as I prefer to follow a "better safe than sorry" philosophy. "When in doubt, leave it out" is a great rule of thumb, and it is what I do.
- **Bone Broth** (*Note: this should be homemade. Search online for a recipe. This is NOT the same thing as bouillons or canned broths, which should be avoided. You also don't want to drink this all day long. Have one cup and move on.*)
- **1 or 2 teaspoons of heavy cream** (*Note how little this amount is! Even so, you should not drink cup after cup with heavy cream over the course of your day, as it will add up over time and will keep you from burning your own fat. Have ONE cup, with 1 or 2 teaspoons MAX, per day. Personally, I find that heavy cream, even in small amounts, makes me hungry. My best advice is to learn to like your coffee black. If I can do it, YOU can do it.*)
- **A little coconut oil** (*This is a tweak that a lot of people in the intermittent fasting community enjoy, but just like with cream, it makes me hungrier. I also have the philosophy that I would rather be burning the fat from my body than the fat from my coffee cup, so I avoid anything like this during the fast.*)

<u>Probably NOT okay to have during the fast: to be safe, avoid these things:</u>

- **Fruity and sweet flavored teas** (*even if the label says "0 calories" and no sweeteners are listed*)
- **Flavored coffees** (*as with the teas—these can taste very sweet. Do you want to risk spiking your insulin for some "cinnamon roll" flavored coffee? NO, YOU DO NOT.*)
- **Fruit flavored sparkling waters**
- **Gum** (even sugarless)
- **Breath mints** (even sugarless)

<u>For-the-Love-of-God and without question, do NOT have during the fast!</u>

- **Products containing artificial sweeteners**, such as aspartame (NutraSweet), saccharine, and sucralose (Splenda)
- **Diet sodas**
- **"Diet" ANYTHING**
- **Stevia** (even though it may be marketed as "natural")
- **Sugar alcohols** (xylitol, erythritol, most things ending with –ol, etc.)
- **Any sweeteners that I forgot to mention** (*even if they develop a new "miracle" sweetener. Just NO. Sweet=NO. No matter what they tell you about it. No.*)
- **Bouillon**
- **Canned or store-bought broths**
- **Food of any type,** even if it is "0 calorie." (*If you have to chew it, you shouldn't have it during the fast...other than ice. Chew ice at your own risk, though...your dentist told me to tell you that.*)
- **Coffee creamers of any kind** (*this includes substitute milks such as almond milk, which for some reason, people seem to think should be allowed, but aren't*)

I'm sure there are other things you shouldn't have that I haven't thought of. Here is a great rule of thumb: If you ever aren't sure about something, ask yourself this: does it taste sweet or have calories? If the answer is yes, don't try to squeeze it into your fast or rationalize it. If the answer is "I am not sure," then treat it as a yes and avoid it.

Remember: I already said that you don't have to worry about occasional tooth brushing or use of mouthwash. Yes, those products may contain some sort of sweetener. Yes, those products may have a sweet taste. But you are only using them for a moment, so brush, swish, and be done with it.

People have a REALLY HARD TIME giving up their favorite things from the lists above. As I mentioned, I really fought myself on the stevia until I took a hard look at what I was doing to myself.

We all know that in any typical diet, there are usually "free foods." Pickles. Diet Jell-O. Plain popcorn. All of these are "low-calorie." There is even a train of thought in the fasting community that if you are having fewer than 50 calories, you don't "break the fast." Based on my research, I reject that philosophy. To me, "free foods" smack of "diet thinking," and my recommendation is to stop trying to work in added items during the fast. The only things you should have during the fast are the items I specified earlier: water, black coffee, plain tea, and various fizzy waters, all unflavored and unsweetened.

From experience, let me share this very important piece of advice. I have been in a lot of diet and weight loss groups over the years, most of which were on Facebook. It's a great way to connect with people who have common interests, and these groups can be a fantastic support system. Do you know what the most common thing I hear from people in these groups about diet sodas/stevia/creamers/flavored coffees? "It's okay—they don't affect MY weight loss."

People are in denial about their beloved sweet, creamy, and flavored products. Just because they have lost some weight, they assume that everything is working just fine. And then, these same people never seem to be able to lose the last few pounds to get to goal, or they get to goal briefly and then have rebound weight gain. (In fact, rebound weight gain is the biggest problem that I see from these people.) The heavy diet soda/flavored coffee/sweetener users NEVER have results as good as the people who avoid the artificial sweeteners during the fast. They also struggle more with hunger and compliance, because their satiety signals don't get into balance as easily. These people are stuck in the CI/CO mindset, where it is only about the calories. When you understand how insulin works to lock away your fat stores, you completely understand why it's counterproductive to include products that will spike your insulin during the fast.

Remember this: if you try to get away with having the forbidden items, you are only cheating yourself. You may think you are losing weight just fine, but you aren't really accessing your fat as effectively as you could be, because of the constant release of insulin. Instead of reaping the beneficial hormonal effects of the fast, you are actually causing hormonal damage—you just can't see it.

Chapter 11

Intermittent fasting is a lifestyle, not a religion

Intermittent fasting is a lifestyle rather than just another diet, and you have to follow it consistently in order to get results. It isn't something you do until you lose the excess weight; rather, it's something that you will want to continue permanently. Not only does intermittent fasting allow you to maintain your loss effortlessly, but it also provides so many other health benefits that I covered in the chapter about why you should consider fasting. As an example, my inflammation has gone down so much that I don't even need daily allergy medication anymore—even in peak pollen season (and if you have ever been to Augusta, GA during the Masters Golf Tournament, when pollen is at its peak, you'll know that it is not unusual to see drifts of yellow pollen blowing in the streets).

When I dabbled in intermittent fasting from 2009-2014, I never could convince myself that it was something I wanted to—or could—do forever. I was caught up in the mentality that you "dieted" only until you reached your weight loss goal, and then you magically maintained the loss, forever and ever, amen. When I finally realized that there was no actual finish line, and weight maintenance would take some level of change for the rest of my life, I accepted that intermittent fasting was the ONLY way I could see myself living my life forever.

Once you choose an intermittent fasting plan to begin, you'll have to figure out how to make it work for you. There is nothing wrong in trying different approaches. Read over the examples I provided in the book, and also consider reading the original books that I have listed in the annotated bibliography. Each of those books goes into the plans in much more detail than I have here.

So why do I say that intermittent fasting is a lifestyle and "not a religion"? It's because I want you to forgive yourself when life gets in your way. You will take a day off to live your life, and that's okay. You'll have a vacation, or a holiday, and you'll want to turn your eating window into a revolving door. Trust me—I do that, too. You do NOT have to be perfect every single day for intermittent fasting to work.

Really understand that last sentence: you do NOT have to be perfect, no matter which intermittent fasting plan you choose. If you take a day off, you don't need to repent of your sins, or feel like you have failed.

The key is this: you are living a lifestyle. LIVING. Life is messy and imperfect, despite your best intentions. Sometimes we feast, and sometimes we fast. Feasting doesn't mean you are weak—it means you are human.

Let me give you some examples of how I have lived this lifestyle this year. I went on TWO cruises this summer. One was for five days with my husband to celebrate our 25th anniversary. Then, less than a week later, I went on a 4-day cruise with my best friends from college. What are cruises known for? If you said FOOD, you would be right. And guess what—I didn't fast while I was on the cruise ships. I did skip breakfast most days, and I didn't start eating until lunchtime most days, but I definitely ate at least 2 full meals each day, plus there were trips to the buffet for an afternoon (or late night) snack. I had a regular food-baby by the time I got off of the ship—particularly the second cruise. I didn't want to eat a big meal for a long time after that.

I no longer weigh myself, so I have no idea what my weight did after all of that feasting. I do know that my clothes were tight when I got off of the second ship, but within a week I felt back to normal. I got right back to my fasting routine like the trips never even happened, and my body sorted itself out. There was no guilt, and I didn't have to do any sort of penance once I got back home.

I also fully embraced feasting over the holidays this year, while still maintaining my fasting lifestyle. We get a week off for Thanksgiving, and there was a LOT of feasting going on at my house. My older son was home from college, and his girlfriend also stayed with us for the week. I was constantly preparing some sort of meal for someone—waffles for breakfast, delicious lunches, full dinners. I didn't eat breakfast on any of the days, but there were definitely days where I ate lunch and dinner. And Thanksgiving was one big food-fest. Still, I balanced the days of feasting with days that included shorter windows. I felt really full when I went back to work on the Monday after Thanksgiving, but within a few days, I felt like myself again. When I measured my waist on December 14th, I found that I had lost an inch in my waist from the time I had measured one month prior, on November 14th. I was able to balance out the feasting with fasting.

Of course, don't forget about Christmas! If you are like me, the holiday revolves around food and parties. Parties are easy—most of the time, they are in my window. Since my motto is "delay, don't deny," I can eat whatever I want once my window is open, with zero guilt. The more difficult times are when food is constantly available—such as the continual influx of treats. As a teacher, students start bringing me sweet treats in early December. I have learned how to save them until I get home, and if I want something, I'll eat it in my window.

Some days, though, you do want to relax and fully embrace the festivities. I decided to do that on the last day of school before Christmas break. It's a half-day for students, and we always have a luncheon for the teachers and staff. I debated passing on the luncheon, but instead decided to fully embrace the day as the food fest it could be. To be honest—I really miss one thing while fasting, and that is breakfast from Chick-fil-a. If you aren't familiar with that particular fast food restaurant, I am sorry for you. It's a staple here in the south. You can't get their breakfast any time other than breakfast hours, Monday-Saturday (because they don't open on Sunday). I decided that I WOULD eat a chicken biscuit meal that day. And I would eat the sweet treats. And I would eat the lunch. And then I would eat dinner that night. Sigh. I felt gross by 9 a.m., and I was already tired of eating. You'll be glad to know that I persevered, and by the end of the day, I had completely gotten feasting out of my system. Call it a "metabolic boost" day, and then move on.

Sometimes, we need days like that one to remind us of why we choose to fast. I was completely ready to hop back into my intermittent fasting routine the next day. It was a relief, actually. Feast, and then fast. I feel so much better following an intermittent fasting lifestyle than I do when I eat all day long. Shockingly better. So much better, in fact, that I know I will never revert to my old eating habits.

That one day of overdoing it actually helped me stay somewhat on track on Christmas Eve and Christmas Day. On Christmas Eve I stuck to a 6-hour window, and on Christmas Day I gave myself an 8-hour window. I just didn't feel like overdoing it again. I ate whatever looked good, but I closed my window before I felt stuffed or miserable. For the next couple of days, I naturally didn't want to eat much. In fact, both days I got busy and didn't open my window until after 6 p.m. My satiety hormones told me that I didn't need to eat much, and it was nice to listen.

Two days after Christmas, I decided to try on my honesty pants. You know what I mean—there are some items of clothing that have absolutely zero stretch, and these items will never lie to you about your weight. I have two pairs of these honesty pants, and they slipped right on, buttoning easily with no muffin-top. I think they actually felt better than they did when I tried them on early in the fall.

The reason I told you about all of my debauchery on the cruises, over Thanksgiving, and at Christmas was to illustrate that I am not a perfect intermittent faster. Intermittent fasting is my lifestyle, yes. I follow it almost every day. BUT—I take time to live my life when I decide that it is worth it. There are special occasions like vacations and the celebrations of life where you will decide to feast, and not fast. As long as you make intermittent fasting your lifestyle, it's okay. After all, fasting is a lifestyle, not a religion.

Chapter 12

Saturday is not a special occasion
(*It happens every week...*)

In the last chapter, I discussed how it is not only fine to deviate from your intermittent fasting plan on occasion, it is part of life. We aren't in a religious cult, after all.

HOWEVER...

You need to carefully define what is actually a special occasion in your life.

A family vacation: that is clearly a special occasion. A major holiday: definitely a special occasion. A weekly Sunday lunch at your family member's house: sorry, that's NOT a special occasion, because it happens every week (although you could totally make it work within your eating window or with your up day schedule, and still be on plan).

When something happens frequently in your life, such as a weekly business meeting that involves food, that is a part of your lifestyle. For anything that is a part of your regular lifestyle, keep it in mind when planning your fasting regimen, and most definitely plan your fasting schedule around these regularly occurring events. It's the infrequent occurrences that are special occasions.

In order to be successful, you need to design your intermittent fasting schedule so that it accommodates the way you want to live your regular life. True special occasions should be rare, and you don't want to impulsively decide to abandon your intermittent fasting plan at every whim. That's a slippery slope, and before you know it, your fasting is so intermittent that you are no longer on any plan at all. Ask me how I know... (The years 2009-2014 from my own life come to mind.)

Chapter 13

We don't cheat—we PLAN

I want you to remove one word from your vocabulary, and that word is "cheat." You aren't married to intermittent fasting, so you can't cheat on it.

That may sound like a joke, but I'm serious. Words are powerful. We would all agree that the idea of cheating has a negative connotation in every context. You cheat on a diet; you don't cheat on a lifestyle.

Sometimes people ask if they can have a "cheat day," and of course, the answer is NO, because we don't use the word "cheat." If you remember the story I told a couple of chapters ago about the day before Christmas break, you recall that was a pretty epic day of feasting. But— understand that it was fully planned. I made a choice to indulge myself, and I did it. There was zero guilt.

This is the important distinction: cheating is always a bad thing. When you cheat on something or someone you feel guilty about it. In our intermittent fasting lifestyle, we never cheat, so we don't have to feel guilt about what we eat. Ever. YOU ARE IN CONTROL. Period. Own it.

When you make a plan to indulge, you should fully savor every bite of food. For one special and unusual day, you may choose to eat in a hedonistic style that is atypical. You EMBRACE that planned indulgence. You also notice that you probably don't feel very well by the end of the day. You pay attention to the signals your body sends you. While you don't feel guilt, you probably DO feel uncomfortable, and it helps you realize that days like this are unusual in your life for a reason.

I have mentioned my Facebook group several times, and it's so interesting to see the posts members share after a holiday. We are universally ready to get back into our fasting routines after a day or two of planned feasting. Because we openly discuss our indulgences, with zero guilt attached, we understand that it is fine to include these feasting days as a part of an intermittent fasting lifestyle. We intellectually know that these days should be few and far between, and we also acknowledge that we feel better when we follow our fasting routine.

We don't ever cheat, but we do have occasional planned indulgences. Big difference.

Chapter 14

To weigh, or not to weigh? That is the question

Many people ask how much weight they can expect to lose when following an intermittent fasting lifestyle. I can't possibly answer that question, because it depends on so many different factors.

First of all, you need to understand that intermittent fasting is not a fast weight loss plan. You may be one of the lucky few who lose 10 pounds in one week (very rare, but it happens), or you might gain weight in the first week or two and think this plan doesn't work. Realistically, once your body adjusts to intermittent fasting, a pound per week is a steady rate of loss. Keep your expectations realistic, and don't expect to lose all of your excess weight at a fast pace. Your body may need to heal some underlying hormonal issues first, before it's ready to release pounds. Give yourself time, and be patient. Many people find that they lose inches before they lose pounds.

So what about weighing? The scale—love it or hate it, it's a fixture for most dieters. We have all been on diets where we stand before the scale, crossing our fingers, hoping to see a certain number. We exhale, and step on...

What happens next depends on the number. If it is lower, we feel victorious! We are mastering this whole business of weight loss!

What, though, if the number is…HIGHER????!?! Horrors! What a failure. A higher number on the scale can ruin your whole day.

What if I told you that weight loss is rarely linear, and that the scale is a terrible day-to-day measure of whether you are losing fat or not? So many things affect what that scale tells you. Maybe you are retaining water from the pizza you ate last night. Perhaps you are experiencing hormonal monthly weight gain (that one is strictly for the ladies…). Realistically, you can't expect to see your weight go down, down, down, day after day. If you do expect that, you will not only be disappointed, you will think you are a failure.

I have read a theory that explains what may happen in your body when you lose fat, but the scale refuses to budge. Google "Of Whooshes and Squishy Fat" to read the fascinating explanation in depth. It's a classic blog post that I have seen people refer to for years as an explanation of what may be happening when we are losing fat but not registering a loss on the scale. To briefly summarize the theory, your fat cells may hold onto water as a part of the fat loss process. You're gradually losing fat, but your body replaces the fat with water, which means you don't lose any weight on the scale. This can continue for days and days at a time, if not a week or more. Then, suddenly, WHOOSH! You seemingly lose several pounds overnight. This happens because your body released the water it had been storing in your fat cells all at once, resulting in that sudden drop on the scale. This is a theory, and as far as I know it hasn't been scientifically proven; however, I have been in enough weight loss groups in my day to know that the "whoosh" effect is real, and many people experience it.

So, now that we understand that the scale can be a terrible measure of what is happening in your body day-to-day, you probably want to know: should we weigh daily? Weekly? Monthly? Never? The answer is this: it depends

on YOU, and how the scale makes you feel. If one bad
weight reading will make you feel defeated, causing you to
reject intermittent fasting entirely, then you should be on
team no-weigh. If, however, you can take an objective look
at the daily measurement and go on about your day with no
self-judgment, then you are someone who can handle
weighing.

While actively losing, I weighed daily. Then, once per
week (every Friday), I calculated the average of the past 7
days. (For the math-phobic among us, it's a simple
calculation: add the 7 weights and divide by 7. If you only
have 6 weights, you add them and divide by 6. You have
my permission to use a calculator.)

Each week, I only compared the weekly averages.
There were some weeks where my Friday-to-Friday weight
was UP, but my weekly average was ALWAYS down. Let's
take a look at how that looked for me:

	Sunday	Monday	Tuesday	Wed.	Thur.	Friday	Weekly Average
4	185.1	184.2	184.9	185.2	185.3	185.0	185.1	185.0
4 4	185.9	184.1	184.2	184.2	184.1	183.3	184.0	184.2
4 4	184.1	184.4	184.1	182.9	182.4	182.2	183.0	183.3
14	183.8	183.2	183.8	183.1	183.0	183.9	182.5	183.3
14	183.6	183.2	183.0	183.4	182.4	181.9	182.8	182.9
14 14	182.5	183.2	182.5	181.9	180.8	180.7	179.3	181.6
14 14	178.7	178.0	178.2	177.8	178.4	178.9	180.3	178.6
14 14	178.6	177.8	178.4	177.4	178.1	179.3	177.7	178.1
14)/14	177.7	176.9	177.9	175.8	175.9	176.4	175.4	176.5
1/14- 7/14	174.7	176.6	176.6	177.3	176.5	175.2	176.3	176.2
3/14- 4/14	176.6	177.9	177.0	174.7	172.5	170.9	169.6	174.1 —

73

That is a photo of my (very old-school) weight record from the fall of 2014. The quality is terrible, and I wasn't planning on sharing it with the world, but I want to dig into some of the data from the photo with you. If you go down the list of Friday weights, you see it goes like this: 185.1, 184.0, 183.0, 182.5, 182.8…WAIT! My Friday weight went UP that week. Had the plan stopped working??? Was I gaining weight?

If I was only weighing weekly, I could have mistakenly thought I was, indeed, gaining weight. The weekly averaging saved my sanity. When I compared the weekly average from that week (in the highlighted column), I saw that the average had been 183.3 the week before, but this week's average was 182.9. My weekly average was down by almost half a pound. That's not much, but it is downward movement.

Two weeks later, it happened again. One Friday I was 179.3, and then the following Friday I weighed in at 180.3. Did I gain a pound that week???

Thank you, weekly averaging, for telling me the true story. When I look at the weekly averages for those two weeks, I see that the first weekly average was 181.6, and the second was 178.6. I didn't GAIN a pound that week! On the contrary: my weekly average went DOWN by 3 pounds. It was a GREAT week, not a failure.

This is not a fast process, and weight loss is rarely linear. Trust the process, and if you weigh, weigh daily and only compare weekly averages. These days I don't weigh at all, and it feels much better to me. I stick to my intermittent fasting lifestyle, and I trust the process. My clothes tell the story, and as they slowly get looser, I know I am losing fat. Tight pants that are getting looser tell the story much better than the scale. NEVER let the scale convince you this isn't working if your clothes are telling another story.

Chapter 15

What should I EAT? Delay, Don't Deny!

The title of this book is *Delay, Don't Deny*, and this is not the chapter where I reveal that you have to actually eat in some special way in order for intermittent fasting to work. I legitimately do not deny myself of anything that I want to eat. I do, however, delay when I eat. I delay so I don't have to deny! It's so very freeing.

Before settling happily into an intermittent fasting lifestyle, I tried every single diet plan that promised that you could eat "as much as you want" as long as you avoided certain things. Those plans never resulted in any long-lasting weight loss for me. I tried it all: low fat, high fat, low carb, high carb, gluten-free, vegetarian, all-natural, organic, etc. There was no magical plan where I could eat as much as I wanted to eat (within their guidelines) and lose weight.

No, I am not going to tell you what you can and can't eat. I assume that if you are reading this book, you are an adult, and you understand that some foods are more nutritious than others. You know that your body needs nutrients in order to function. Some foods have more nutrients than others, and you want to make sure that your diet includes a variety of these nutrients for optimal health. Vegetables, nutrients. Jelly beans, no nutrients.

No, I don't restrict any foods specifically within my eating window, but I do make choices based on how foods make me feel. If I open my window with a sugary latte from everyone's favorite coffee chain, I get shaky within a matter of minutes from the sudden hit of sugar into my system. That doesn't mean that I can't have a latte ever again; it just means that I don't choose to open my window with one because I know how it will make me feel. Highly processed foods all make me feel that way when I open my window with them. I can have a cookie, but I shouldn't start with a cookie. I should delay the cookie, in fact.

Do I still eat highly processed foods? Yes. I had Doritos on Christmas day, because they were around and I love them. I know that they are not a nutritious choice; in fact, they are among the most non-nutritive substances on the planet. That's okay, as they don't make up the majority of my regular diet. As I already mentioned, I delay, so I don't have to deny. There are very few things that I absolutely won't eat on principle based on them being "bad foods." (Artificial sweeteners and fake fats are two of the things I won't touch for any reason, ever. I use real sugar, and real fats, such as butter and heavy cream. In fact, I use a LOT of butter and heavy cream. One time my teenage son asked if all of that butter was just for me. Yes, son, it is. Get your own butter. Margarine? NEVAAAAH!!!!!)

I want to share this with you: since following an intermittent fasting lifestyle, I have become a food snob. It's true. I care a lot more about what I put into my body now, and I don't eat something just because it is there. I am more aware of how foods make me feel, and I am actually enjoying high-quality foods more than junk foods.

Many intermittent fasters discover this same thing about themselves. We realize that food becomes something to be savored, and we don't want to "waste" our meals on garbage. Do I eat pizza? Yes. I love pizza. I eat it frequently. But now that I am an intermittent faster, I am more likely to hold out for high-quality pizza rather than settle for a frozen grocery store pizza. (In fact, I would never settle for a frozen grocery store pizza now. Not because I think they are "bad" for me, but because I would rather eat high-quality pizza. It tastes better and makes me happier. I am worth high-quality pizza, darn it!) I won't eat Cool-Whip, but I will eat real whipped cream. I won't eat fat-free cheese, but I will eat full-fat cheese. I don't drink diet sodas, but I'll have a real Coke if I want one. I ALWAYS choose the highest quality foods that are delicious. Every time. Or, I wait and eat later if the food choices are not to my liking. I delay, rather than deny. I am absolutely willing to not eat at all, rather than settle for something that isn't going to be delicious and satisfying.

Would it be better for me to avoid all processed foods and only eat foods that are presented the way nature intended? Sure it would. I have no doubt. There are some very compelling arguments against processed foods, particularly highly refined grains and sugars. However, I have tried to live that way, and I feel overly restricted by the limitations. A life without white flour or sugar? No cookies, or cake, EVER again? No DORITOS? No, thank you. I'd rather have a shorter eating window and eat what makes me happy. Delay, Don't Deny.

So, is it wrong to watch what you eat when you are an intermittent faster? Absolutely not. You can be an intermittent faster and eat according to ANY preferred eating style! Intermittent fasting plus low carb? Check! Intermittent fasting plus vegan? Sure! Intermittent fasting plus all organic? Great choice! Intermittent fasting plus the standard American diet? Go for it! The tool of intermittent fasting works with ANY eating style. (As long as you follow the guidelines for what to ingest during the fast, obviously. If you are spiking your insulin during the fast, all bets are off.)

If you do want to clean up your diet and avoid overly processed foods, you'll assuredly be healthier than I am, and one of the best books I read about avoiding processed foods is *The Science of Skinny*. The author also recommends that you eat frequently throughout the day, which I do not suggest, obviously—but her food recommendations are fantastic. If you are interested in moving toward fewer processed foods, start by reading her book. I'm not going to eat that way, because there is too much "denying" for me, but if you are interested, check it out.

One more subject that needs to be addressed: alcohol. Can alcohol be part of an intermittent fasting lifestyle? Yes, but BE CAREFUL.

First of all, be cautious about opening your window with alcohol. After a period of fasting, the alcohol will go straight to your bloodstream, and you will feel the effects very quickly. For best results, have food with your drinks.

Even so, be careful. (I have said that TWICE, so you know I mean it.) I went to a party about a month ago, and I didn't really have a lot to drink, but I also was busy socializing, and I didn't have much to eat, either. The alcohol went straight to my system, and it wasn't pretty. Always have plenty of food if you are drinking, and understand that you can't drink as much as you used to be able to drink. When intermittent fasting, you are now a cheap drunk, and it's important to recognize that, to avoid your spouse having to place the trashcan beside the bed. Not that that happened to me. This is a completely hypothetical story. And, I will never drink bourbon again. Oops.

As with food, intermittent fasting has also made me a snob when it comes to what I'll drink. I have one perfect glass of prosecco with dinner most nights. One, not two. I could have two if I wanted two—but I don't want two. One seems to be enough for me. I listen to my body, and I don't overdo it. (As a side note, I read an article that said that one glass of champagne or prosecco a day will prevent Alzheimer's, and even if it's a fake story, I choose to embrace it in principle.)

One other note about alcohol. If you are trying to lose weight, alcohol may not be your friend. I've read that our bodies burn off the alcohol first, and so that may affect your weight loss. In addition, your inhibition is lower when drinking, and you may eat more and over a longer period of time than you would have without the alcohol. When I was in weight loss mode, I avoided alcohol completely for a short period of time until I met certain weight loss goals. I drank WATER one New Year's Eve, in fact—and you know how much I love champagne!

Chapter 16

Let's talk about maintenance

I have been in many diet groups over the years, and people seem to struggle with weight regain. We all know the statistics. Something like fewer than 5% of dieters are able to maintain a weight loss.

I have good news! I believe we have found the secret to an effortless maintenance. It's this: keep doing what you are doing. Boom. Done.

As long as we maintain our fasting regimen with consistency, and keep from spiking insulin during the fast, our bodies should happily maintain our ideal weight. The Herrings (Bert, who created the Fast 5 plan, and his wife) found through surveying long time fasters that maintenance was not an issue with those who stick to their recommended 5-hour daily eating window long term. Krista Varady found the same thing in her *Every Other Day Diet* research. Those who maintain a fasting schedule are able to easily maintain their weight loss over a long period of time. (And in *The Every Other Day Diet*, the maintenance fasting schedule is not every other day, thank goodness. You still fast, but not as frequently.)

Ever since I gave up stevia in my coffee, I have had zero trouble with weight regain. (Prior to giving up stevia, I did struggle with about 8 pounds of regain, but ever since I cut it out during the fast, my clothes have just continued to get looser month after month.)

When I look back at the various diet groups I have been in over the years, and I think of the people who keep having to go back to heavily restricting to re-lose the weight they keep regaining, I think there are two common problems. One is the use of flavored/sweet "zero calorie" products during the fasting period. They all claim it "works" for them, but I would argue that if it works, why do you have to keep losing the same 10-20 pounds over and over again?

The other common problem is that people see goal as a finish line, and when they get there, they can "go back to a normal life." I have news for you—there is no finish line. Fasting is a lifestyle—and there's a reason for that. As a lifestyle, if we continue to follow it most days, we will succeed at keeping our bodies balanced hormonally and weight maintenance is a breeze. If we go back to eating frequently most days, we will be in the same hormonal mess that caused us to gain weight in the first place. The lifestyle that caused you problems in the past will cause you problems again if you return to it.

So—the good news is that you can maintain your weight loss if you keep up some sort of fasting regimen. You can experiment to figure out what works for you as a maintenance lifestyle. For me, I need to keep to a pretty consistent routine with not very many planned indulgences. Fortunately, that is easy. The bad news is that you will never be "done" and you won't be returning to your prior eating schedule. It didn't work for you then, and it won't suddenly start working for you now.

As I mentioned in a previous chapter, you CAN be flexible when you need to, for special occasions. You already know that I went on two cruises last summer, and I didn't follow my normal fasting schedule. I did try to delay my first meal of the day as long as possible, but once I opened my window each day, it was OPEN! I fully enjoyed myself on both cruises. When I returned home, my pants were tight—but it only took about a week back on my regular fasting schedule for my body to go back to normal.

As long as I keep to the fast as recommended (without spiking insulin during the day), and I continue an intermittent fasting lifestyle, maintenance is actually easy. I hope that you find the same to be true for you!

Chapter 17

Sharing intermittent fasting with others

To share, or not to share? The more intermittent fasting is understood as a legitimate approach to health and weight loss, the more open people will be to hearing about it. That being said, there are decades of bad dietary advice that must be unlearned first. Not everyone is ready to hear about intermittent fasting.

Here's a fun experiment. Go up to someone and tell them that you never eat until dinner and then you only eat one meal per day, or tell them that three times per week you fast completely. They will probably tell you that you are likely in starvation mode RIGHT NOW, that you MUST eat six small meals every day to protect your metabolism, and then they will worry that you might have an eating disorder. I have gotten that lecture many times. Most of the people who have lectured me are either heavier now than they were when they first criticized fasting, or they are now intermittent fasters themselves. (Nothing will win people over to your "crazy" way of thinking like success. Suddenly, you're not so crazy, and they want to learn more.)

Here's the funny part. NO ONE ever lectured me when I weighed 210 pounds. No one told me that I was harming myself by eating so much food. It's only when I began skipping meals that I started to get pushback from people.

It's okay to keep fasting to yourself if you don't want to talk about it with others. When people are asking you how you are losing weight, tell them that you are watching what you eat. That's true. If people ask why you aren't eating at any particular moment, tell them that you plan to eat later. That's also true. It is really none of their business what you eat or don't eat. I have also found that most people won't even notice that you aren't eating. I went to a party once where no one knew I was fasting. I drank water only, and not one person asked me why I wasn't eating. They were all too drunk to care (I am mostly kidding…). The point is that no one noticed I was drinking ice water and that I didn't eat.

There are some occasions where it's harder to hide what you are doing. If everyone at your workplace eats lunch together, and you suddenly stop eating lunch, they are going to notice. People will definitely comment on what you are doing, and there may be a great deal of pressure from others to eat. I, too, faced that pressure. I remember one particular lunch in the teacher's workroom. I sat there drinking my water, and two different people tag-teamed me about how I should be eating. They were relentless. If I had any doubts about fasting, it would have been hard to deal with the pressure from them. Fortunately for me, I am very confident and well-read about fasting, so I stood my ground. Even so, it was immensely irritating. (One of the teachers sent me an apology email later, so it was obvious that I was annoyed.)

There are several ways that you can deal with this type of issue. You can avoid situations where others are eating to keep the focus off of you. (Instead of sitting with others who are eating, work through lunch.) You can convince a friend to fast with you, so you have support from a buddy. (Safety in numbers!) You can even tell them that your "doctor" has you on a time-restricted eating plan. (Hey, I do have a doctorate—I'm "Dr. Stephens," after all!) Or, you can confidently tell people what you are doing and why, and ignore the criticisms. That can be very hard, and it constantly amazes me how other people think that what you are eating is somehow any of their business.

As you probably know, I follow the last suggestion, and I talk openly about fasting. At the age of 47, I no longer feel like I need to get approval from others about my lifestyle choices, and I have a big mouth, so I'll talk about fasting with anyone, at any time. I never feel pressured to eat just because others are eating.

Some intermittent fasters do, however, face immense pressure from others to eat, and not everyone can shake it off like I can. It's usually people who are closest to you who are the food-pushers, like family members or co-workers. Even when people know that you are fasting, they might try to bring you snacks during your fasting time. They genuinely don't understand how "one little bite" will absolutely hurt you. These food-pushers are hard to handle. Remember this: you NEVER have to eat something to please someone else. YOU are in control of your own body. Unless you do have an eating disorder, such as anorexia, or you are at an unhealthily low BMI, you should never eat to please someone else. It is your body, and you have to live in it.

If the person who is pressuring you is someone you love, like a spouse or a parent, you probably do want to help them understand what you are doing, and explain why it's a legitimate approach to wellness. Once I got a very worried text from my stepmother who was concerned about my "starving-fasting," and she was convinced that I had an eating disorder. (No, I had an eating disorder when I took diet pills throughout the early 2000s. I had an eating disorder when I ate garbage constantly. NOW, I have eating sanity. For the first time in my life, my eating is NOT disordered.)

I sent her a copy of *The Obesity Code* to read so that she would understand the science behind fasting. I am not sure that she ever read it, but my dad did. At any rate, I think it reassured her.

My recommendation is that you buy any naysayers a copy of the book you are currently reading, *Delay, Don't Deny*, and hand it to them so that they understand what you are doing, and why. (Heck, I recommend that you buy stacks of my book, and give a copy to everyone you know. What better present for everyone on your Christmas list?)

Some people, particularly mothers of girls, also worry about what signal they are sending to their young girls by fasting. I understand where these moms are coming from. (Fortunately, I have sons, because God knew that I would screw up any daughters.) I agree that mothers particularly need to be careful about what messages we send to our children about food. That could be a whole other book, in fact. *How Not to Screw Up Your Children.* Maybe I will write that one next.

On a serious note, you do want to tread cautiously where your young children are concerned. You don't want to encourage children or teenagers to fast, or to become weight-obsessed. If you feel that you must discuss it with your children, my advice would be to clearly communicate that the body's nutritional needs change once you are an adult and you are finished growing. Focus on the fact that you fast for health and de-emphasize the weight loss component. Always explain that growing bodies need to be fueled more frequently than adult bodies. Then change the subject. Let them see you eat with gusto when you do eat, and they will realize that food isn't something to be feared. The more matter-of-fact you are about it, the better.

Chapter 18

Finding a support group

If you are fasting alone, it can be very difficult, as I mentioned in the last chapter. You may not be confident that what you are doing is healthy, and there are many temptations to eat every single day. People close to you may not understand what you are doing, and you can be tempted to quit out of frustration. I honestly think that was my problem from 2009-2014. No one I knew in real life had ever heard of intermittent fasting, and there was zero support around me. I would start and stop, start and stop, start and stop. Meanwhile, I got fatter and fatter.

When I got serious about taking control of my health in 2014, I turned to Facebook groups for support. I genuinely believe that these groups have made a huge difference to my long-term success. I have learned so very much from others in these communities.

There are many intermittent fasting groups on Facebook, and some are better than others. I have left all of the groups except for two, and those are the ones where I am the group administrator. I had to leave the others, because in every other group people give terrible advice, such as "Diet soda is GREAT during the fast and it works for me!" Sigh.

To combat all of the misinformation, I felt the need to start my own groups where I can put forth a consistent message about fasting best-practices. The more I understood about how the body works, the harder it was for me to sit back and watch people give bad advice to others. Maybe I can't save the world, but I can control the message in my own little part of it. In my groups, we want to make sure that we are giving advice based on research, so people have the greatest chance of success.

Not all Facebook groups are friendly, by the way. I have actually been thrown out of intermittent fasting groups because of my big mouth. Oops. One of the most infamous Facebook groups in the intermittent fasting community preaches that the only reason intermittent fasting works is because you are restricting calories. Don't even say the word "insulin" to them. They won't allow anyone to mention the idea that fasting has certain metabolic and hormonal advantages beyond just the calorie restriction component, and if you do mention something of the sort, first they will ridicule you, and then they will ban you from the group. I lasted 30 minutes in that group before I was banned. I'm not sure how anyone can read the research and not realize that there is so much more going on in the body than just CI/CO, but they are free to practice intermittent fasting with calorie counting if they want to. I'm pretty sure most of them won't be buying my book, and that's okay with me.

If you are interested in following intermittent fasting using the principles I have outlined in this book, I would like to invite you to join one of my Facebook groups for support. Both are closed groups, meaning that your membership must be approved by an administrator before you can join. I am VERY particular about who joins the groups, and if you have a suspicious looking Facebook profile, I will not approve your membership. Suspicious profiles include ones with very intense privacy settings (because I can't tell if you are a real person), and also profiles where you list multi-level marketing or diet companies as your employer. (No, you can't join my Facebook group and try to sell us your amazing body wraps or protein shakes. I am onto your tricks, people. We also don't want you to join our groups and spam us with links to your blog on nutrition.)

If you are interested in joining, and I deny your request (oops), send me a message on Facebook messenger explaining why you want to join and request membership again. If you mention that you have read my book, you are definitely going to be approved for membership, because I know that you are well informed about how to fast properly.

My first group is called "One Meal A Day IF Lifestyle," and it has been active since August of 2015. In just under a year and a half, we have grown to over 3,500 members. It is a fantastic community of intermittent fasters. As you can tell from the group name, it is targeted specifically to people who follow a one meal a day intermittent fasting approach. Here is a link to it:

https://www.facebook.com/groups/OneMeal/

If you are interested in a group targeted more specifically to the concepts outlined in this book, and one that is open to different types of intermittent fasting besides (and including) one meal a day, you should join my second group: "Delay, Don't Deny: Intermittent Fasting Support." This group is for anyone who wants to follow an intermittent fasting lifestyle of any type, whether it is one meal a day, or 4:3, or something else entirely. Here is a link to it:

https://www.facebook.com/groups/DelayDontDeny/

As I mentioned, finding your own support system can be the difference between success and failure. Intermittent fasting can be quite difficult if you feel like you are alone. If you decide to join our intermittent fasting community, I hope to "see" you around!

Chapter 19

Troubleshooting: What if I am not seeing results?

What if you aren't losing weight OR inches, and yes—you are following your selected fasting regimen just as you should, with nothing that spikes insulin during the fasting time?

It's so hard to feel like you are doing everything right, and getting no results. If you aren't having success, something is happening in your body to prevent weight loss.

First, think about this: how long have you been overweight? If you have been struggling with this long-term, you may be severely insulin resistant. That can lead to high circulating insulin ALL DAY LONG, even when fasting properly. If this is true for you, then there are a couple of options. My first suggestion would be to give yourself more time for the benefits of fasting to kick in. It can take a while to repair years of damage. You may feel like you aren't getting results, but actually, some fantastic healing could be going on in your body.

Another question to consider: have you been restricting calories long term, prior to starting your fasting regimen? If so, you may have slowed your metabolism through the long-term calorie restriction. Remember—your body wants to protect you from starvation, so a slowed metabolism is the expected result of a low-calorie diet. Over time, you need fewer and fewer calories just to maintain your weight. If you think this could be true for you, give yourself some time for the metabolic boosting benefits of fasting to kick in. Make sure that you are not continuing to restrict during your eating window. Eventually, your body should get the message that you aren't in a famine, and the fasting period should boost your metabolism, so you are able to lose weight.

If you have given it awhile and you still aren't seeing any progress, it may be time to consider what you are eating. I know—I said that with intermittent fasting you could eat whatever you want, and that works for most people; however, we are all different. Just because 95% of people can eat whatever they want and lose weight with intermittent fasting, you could be part of the 5% that needs to adapt what you eat. Also, I just made up that 95%/5% statistic. Oops. As far as I know, no one has compiled that data yet. Now, that would be an interesting study.

If you have tried—and I mean, really tried—to follow intermittent fasting, and you are sure that you are fasting properly, AND you aren't losing any weight OR inches, my first suggestion would be to eliminate heavily processed foods for a while and see if that makes a difference. As I mentioned in the chapter on what to eat, *The Science of Skinny* does a great job explaining how to avoid processed foods, and why you might want to consider doing so. Hopefully, this will be the only tweak you need. Again, give yourself some time to see if it works for you.

If you still don't see results after sufficient time has passed, then you may need to consider eating according to low carb/high fat (LCHF) principles for a while. This is a step that you may need to take if you are severely insulin resistant or a type 2 diabetic. Dr. Fung talks about the LCHF lifestyle frequently on his blog at Intensive Dietary Management, and in his book *The Obesity Code*. He pairs intermittent fasting with LCHF eating and has gotten phenomenal results with his patients. Again, I am not a doctor, so you shouldn't take medical advice from me;

however, Dr. Fung IS a doctor, so I recommend searching out his work and seeing what he has to say about it. I believe that he even takes on long-distance patients.

By switching to LCHF, over time it may help you bring down your high insulin levels and tap into fat reserves (if that is, indeed, what is keeping you from losing weight). Based on what I have read, I would predict that after a while, you will begin releasing the weight by pairing LCHF with intermittent fasting. And eventually, you may be able to add back carbs slowly once you have reversed the underlying insulin resistance.

I don't suggest this lightly because you know I love carbs, and I can't imagine not eating them. My motto is "delay, don't deny," and I never want to tell anyone that you need to deny yourself anything you want to eat. Some people do seem to need this extra step, though, and I would not be doing you a favor if I didn't mention it.

One other option for healing underlying insulin resistance is longer fasts. Dr. Fung and Jimmy Moore discuss longer fasts in their collaborative work, *The Complete Guide to Fasting*. That book has a heavy LCHF slant, but they also discuss implementation of longer fasts and why you might want to consider them. If you are interested, I suggest that you read their book for more information. Longer fasts should be attempted under the supervision of a health professional who is experienced with fasting protocols.

There are other factors that can affect weight loss, such as medications and stress. If you are taking any medications that are known for causing weight gain, you are probably going to have a harder time losing weight. Of course, do not stop any medications without your doctor's approval. If you are under a great deal of stress, your body can resist weight loss through the actions of excess cortisol. As we learned in the chapter about insulin, hormones are very important in our bodies, and they control many functions behind the scenes. Try to find ways to manage the stress in your life, and make sure you are getting enough sleep. Easier said than done, AmIRight?

Most importantly, if you feel like you aren't getting results, make sure that you really AREN'T getting results. I have seen people who claim they are not getting results, and in actuality, they haven't given themselves enough time, or they have unrealistic expectations. As I mentioned, intermittent fasting isn't a fast weight loss plan. Just because weight loss isn't fast, that doesn't mean that it isn't happening at exactly the right pace for your body. Remember the power of weighing daily and then taking a weekly average for comparison purposes, or throw away the scale completely. Even if you don't see fast results, intermittent fasting has so many other positive effects beyond weight loss.

Chapter 20

A word about exercise

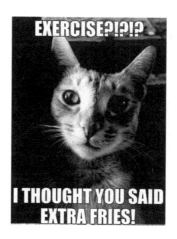

Move. The end. There's your word.

I kid, I kid.

We all know that exercise is good for our bodies. Studies show that exercise helps our mood, as well. But do you know that exercise is not really that effective for weight loss?

Now you probably think I have lost my mind. You have heard all of your life that you need to exercise to lose weight. The more you move your body, the slimmer you will be, right?

I have certainly heard it my whole life: if you want to lose weight, move more. When I was young, the exercise craze was really taking off. Olivia Newton-John wanted to get "Physical." (In hindsight, I am pretty sure that's not what she really meant...even though she was wearing workout clothes in the videos.) Everyone loved Jazzercise. People started to jog. Aerobics classes took off around the country. We were "Sweating to the Oldies." Fast forward to 2016: these days, there is a fitness center on almost every corner. Heck, you can work out 24 HOURS A DAY if you want to!

Has this made us thinner and healthier as a nation? Absolutely not, as I am sure you know.

Time to pull in another study:

http://www.cell.com/current-biology/abstract/S0960-9822(15)01577-8

This study is called "Constrained Total Energy Expenditure and Metabolic Adaptation to Physical Activity in Adult Humans." Do you recognize any words from the Biggest Loser study I mentioned in the chapter on calories? Hopefully, you realize that "metabolic adaptation" is present in the title of this study, as well.

In this 2016 study, researchers expected that as physical activity went up, energy expenditure would go up, as well. It's what we have all been told: move more, burn more. Our portable fitness tracking wristbands tell us precisely how much we are burning at all times, right? Well, the hypothesis did seem to hold true for moderate activity levels when compared to low levels of activity. However, what was not expected is that there appears to be a point where the body adapts, and no further benefits in energy expenditure are realized.

What this means is: people who move moderately do burn more energy than people who are sedentary; however, when you try to ramp up your physical activity beyond "moderate" activity levels, your body adapts and energy expenditure does not increase as expected.

So—should you exercise? Of course, you should! Moderate activity is important for health, and it will provide some benefits with energy expenditure. Find an enjoyable way to move your body. Have fun!

But you do NOT need to do hours and hours of weekly cardiovascular exercise that you don't enjoy. Remember—anything more than "moderate" exercise is not going to make your energy expenditure increase, as your body will adapt.

Excessive exercise always made me hungrier, anyway. Our grandparents called it "working up a good appetite" for a reason.

Exercise for health in a way you enjoy moving your body—but don't think that it is going to make you lose a lot of weight.

As we age, resistance training/weight training/muscle building activities are also useful for overall health. These types of exercise are very good for us, and I highly encourage you to incorporate some sort of muscle building activities into your routine. But will they help us lose weight?

You may have heard that increased muscle mass increases metabolism, and according to my brief research on the topic (I asked Uncle Google), an increase of 2-5 pounds of muscle mass DOES rev up metabolism …by about 50 calories of energy expenditure per day. Get one of those 100 calorie packs of cookies and throw away half of them. Congratulations! You have really earned that half-pack of gross cookies! (On second thought, throw all of them away and eat something that tastes better, like cheesecake. That's what I'd do.)

As with cardio, resistance training is very good for your body, but it isn't going to cause dramatic weight loss for most of us.

I try to move my body in ways that I enjoy. I will take a walk after dinner around the neighborhood with my husband. I have a weighted hula-hoop, and I will use it for a few minutes before bed. (I am AMAZING at the hula-hoop, by the way.)

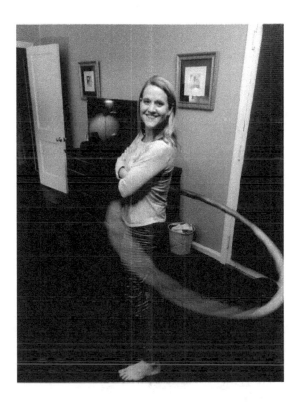

I also own a machine called a vibration plate. It's supposed to be great for working our muscles efficiently. It doesn't take much time to use, and I really enjoy it.

So, about exercise: YES. You totally need to move your body...but don't expect weight loss miracles related to exercise. Exercise for health, not for weight loss.

Appendix A: My weight loss story

I have always been interested in diets, even when I was the skinniest and smallest kid in my class. Growing up, I was scrawny, and I remember being all knobby knees and bony elbows. Even so, I watched my mother, a dance teacher, as she dieted over the years. She had a calorie counting book, and everything you could think of was written in there. (I remember "abalone" was on the first page, and someone had underlined it in pencil. I've never eaten abalone—what even IS it?—but, I remember seeing it in that little book.)

Because of watching my mother count calories, when I packed on the Freshman 15, I decided that the best way to lose a little weight was calorie counting. I cut back for a few weeks, and, BAM! Back to normal. Those were the days, right? It seemed so simple back in my late teens. My weight was fairly constant and I didn't have to think about it much, but whenever I wanted to drop a few pounds, calorie counting worked for me. All throughout college, calorie counting was the method of choice to maintain my desired weight.

There is one funny story that I have to share. During that period, I remember my college roommate and I tried a super-fun diet called the "shot of rice" diet. I think she made it up—I hope so, anyway—the plan was, whenever we got hungry, we would microwave a shot of rice in a small bowl of water, and then we also drank a lot of beer. Hey, it was college. She and I remain great friends to this day, and I was able to introduce HER to intermittent fasting. It is a lot more delicious eating this way than following the shot of rice diet (though there is a lot less beer now).

After I graduated from college and began teaching, I found that the school cafeteria lunches were causing me to pack on the pounds. It was the early 90s, and I weighed maybe 135-140 pounds on a 5' 5" frame. Probably 5 of the pounds were my bangs, and hairspray was my best friend (any ladies my age know of what I speak—if not, Google 1990s hair, and once you stop laughing, you can pick up reading from here). This was the period of time where fat was the enemy, and suddenly there was no more need for calorie counting.

The first diet book I read was the T-Factor Diet, and it sounded awesome. I decided to give it a try. I honestly can't remember what the "T" stands for, but I remember the message of the book: fat makes you fat. That made so much sense. Fat makes you fat! Of course, it does! If you eat fat, it will instantly be deposited on your body. Eat as much food as you want as long as you avoid fat, and you will be THIN! At the time, fat-free was all the rage, and you could buy fat-free everything. Snackwells! Jelly Beans! Potatoes! Corn! All low fat! I would drive through McDonald's on my way to work and order two-fat free apple muffins. It was okay to drink a Coke with it, because Coke is also fat-free. I remember telling my Grandmother about what I was doing and how science-y it was, and she said, in typical Grandmother wisdom, "If corn makes you thin, why do they give it to pigs to fatten them up?"

Of course, I ignored her and went on with my fat gram counting. You know what? I actually lost a little bit of weight, as long as I kept up with the counting and never ate anything that was delicious. Eventually, though, I grew sick of fat-free chocolate covered fat-free marshmallow cookies and fat-free dry potatoes, and realized that I LOVE FAT. Butter, I Love You. No, fat-free was not for me long term.

Next up, calorie counting, part deux. I remembered my early success with calorie counting, and it seemed like the best idea at the time. I was used to counting things, so I would count calories again. I read that 1200 calories per day was the perfect amount for weight loss, so I started counting up everything I ate. My family still makes fun of me for that one time I brought a frozen entrée to a family dinner. I remember what brand of frozen spaghetti I brought, and that it had 220 calories. Counting calories worked for me again, and I got down to a tiny 118 pounds. Eventually, though, I got tired of counting up all of those calories and monitoring every little bite that went into my mouth. Even so, calorie counting remained my go-to strategy for years when I wanted to drop a few (or dozens of) pounds. Of course, it works for a while, but it is miserable to stick to over a long period of time. Not only that, but your body will eventually rebel and your body will adapt. Your metabolism will slow (which I discuss in the chapter about calories and the Biggest Loser study) and, SHAZAM! Weight loss stops, and then the dreaded weight regain begins. Calorie counting wears you down after a while. If you have done it, you know what I mean.

After having my two sons 18 months apart in 1998 and 1999, I needed to lose weight again. I found myself at 163 pounds after the second pregnancy, which was horrifying to me because that was the weight I was when I went into the hospital to deliver my first son. (It doesn't sound all that high NOW, since I eventually topped 210…) One of my friends was losing weight, and I asked her how. Diet pills! Wowza! I could go to the doctor and get a prescription for diet pills that would curb my appetite and I would lose weight? Sign me up for that! So that is exactly what I did. I would absolutely not recommend it to anyone, but it sure worked for me at the time. I was always on edge and I couldn't sleep, but I was THIN again! Finally! As long as I took the magic diet pills, I had no appetite, and I lost weight. I maintained that regimen for more years than I want to admit. I looked great, though. I was able to maintain a size 4-6, and felt great in my own skin—when I didn't feel like I was jumping OUT of my skin, that is. Fortunately, I realized that I was probably doing damage to my body, and I stopped with the diet pills. Of course, my weight rebounded like crazy. I put on 50 pounds in a year and a half. Oops.

After that, I finally read my first low carb diet book. Forget low fat; the science behind low carb eating made perfect sense. Dr. Atkins, you are a genius! I can eat my beloved butter! I can eat it straight from a spoon if I want to! THIS was finally the plan for me! Cheese. Hot dogs. Meat. Bacon. Eggs. STRAIGHT HEAVY CREAM in my coffee! Gag. Knowing what I know now from reading *The Obesity Code*, I know why I wasn't successful at low carb eating (protein also spikes insulin), but I sure gave it a try... over, and over, and over again. I was never able to last more than a week or two before I would cave. I remember one time standing at the kitchen pantry shoving those fried onions (that you put on a green bean casserole) straight into my mouth. My body was crying out for some carbs. I never felt well eating low carb, and I also never got that sense of well-being that some low-carb eaters describe. I always felt like I was STARVING.

From 2005-2008, I bounced from low carb to low calorie, always trying to keep my weight in control. Unfortunately, my weight continued to spiral up and up and up. I gave up for a while and started ignoring the problem. And I bought bigger pants. And bigger pants. And still bigger pants. My former size 6 pants looked like doll's clothes to me, and I was busting out of a size 16. I was dieting myself bigger and bigger every year.

My next foray into dieting was hCG. I heard about it from a friend, who heard about it from her dentist, or something like that. It was a super-secret diet from the 50s, based on the work of a "famous European weight loss doctor," and you injected yourself with pregnancy hormone (hCG) daily to "trick" your body into thinking you were pregnant. The premise is that our bodies are protected by hCG while pregnant, and even if we are starving, our bodies want us to produce a healthy baby; therefore, our metabolisms won't slow even though we are eating only 500 calories a day for 6 weeks. Oh, did I forget to mention that part? You have to eat 500 calories a day for 6 weeks from a very short list of "allowed" foods, and you also inject yourself with hCG that may or may not come from the urine of pregnant mares. Yes, I was officially that desperate. I injected myself with what-might-have-been-mare-pee, and I was able to lose weight. The weight just fell off at the rate of about ½ a pound per day. Well, of course, it did—I was eating 500 calories of food per day. When my 40th birthday rolled around in 2009, I was at a nice weight for me. I fit into a size 8, and I KNEW that hCG was the miracle I had always been looking for. Not so fast. The rebound weight gain from THAT plan was insane. I was unable to keep the weight off and got more and more desperate.

It was at that point that I discovered the key to weight loss—intermittent fasting—only I wasn't ready for it yet. I can't remember which book I found first: it was either *Fast 5*, or *The Alternate-Day Diet*. Instinctually, I knew that intermittent fasting would be my answer. The problem was that I still lived with a diet mentality. I would halfheartedly try fasting for a week or two, and then quit. I felt like I "deserved" to eat all day, just like everyone else. I wasted so many years, with the answer right in my grasp. You know what—I'm not sorry about it. I think I NEEDED to become obese to appreciate how magical it feels to be slim. If I had never become obese, I may have settled for being merely overweight for the rest of my life. Thank you, obesity, for slapping me in the face and making me see the light.

From 2009-2014, I dabbled in various intermittent fasting plans interspersed with more and more desperate diet attempts. These were the years where I bought every diet book and tried it, and I bought every weight loss supplement ever sold. Shakes, pills, cleanses...I tried them all. Every multi-level marketing plan that exists? Again...I tried them all. The shakes were literally the WORST. I remember one plan where you were supposed to have a shake for breakfast, and a shake for lunch, and then a "sensible dinner." All those shakes did was make my stomach mad, and I was STARVING. All. The. Time. Those shakes cost hundreds of dollars per month, and I didn't get thin. What a waste of time and money.

My ultimate wake-up call came in April of 2014. I was on a cruise with my family, and I can remember how tired I was. We were hiking the trails in Belize, and climbing the Mayan ruins, and I could barely move my big body up the steps. Then, I saw myself in a photo. Who WAS that? I looked like someone had inflated my body with an air pump. At that very moment, I hit rock bottom, and decided that I would NOT be that obese woman any longer. Nope.

Here I am in front of the Mayan ruins in Belize with my husband. I didn't feel like I was in the right body; it was hard moving through the day while carrying that much excess weight.

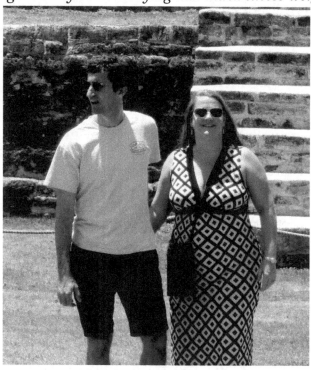

When we got back from that trip, I was officially done with obesity, and it was like a switch had been flipped. I was ready to take my life back. I turned to my trusty friend: hCG. This time, I found a local clinic that was incredibly expensive, because I knew that if I spent a lot of money, I would be committed. I was right. Every day, I would inject myself with hCG, and I would eat my 500 calories. Weigh-ins at the clinic were once a week, and the accountability of those weigh-ins kept me from giving up. The guy who weighed us in was young, and I was NOT going to be the fat lady who didn't lose weight. NOPE. I lost 25 pounds in 5 weeks, and started to feel better.

After a round of hCG, we were expected to take a "maintenance break" for 6 weeks before we could do another round. At that point, I fully intended to hCG-myself down to goal. During the maintenance break, we were required to eat low carb foods only, and we couldn't eat any "sugars or starches." We were also expected to weigh daily, and if our weight ever went up more than 2 pounds from our baseline number, we had to have a "steak day": we were expected to abstain from food all day, and then eat a HUGE steak for dinner. Nothing with the steak; just the steak. Isn't that crazy?

I kept to the low carb plan for the full 6 weeks, and decided that low carb actually made a lot of sense. I re-read *Good Calories, Bad Calories*, and decided that this time, low carb WAS going to be the plan for me. I vowed that I would never go back to that hCG clinic for another round of madness; I was DONE with that crazy restrictive plan. The science behind low carb made so much sense, and I threw myself into the LCHF/Keto community fully. I joined all of the Facebook groups, and I bought all of the books. I was in it to win it! The science was very compelling: insulin causes us to gain weight, and we need to lower our insulin to lose weight. Does that sound familiar?

Unfortunately, I never lost any weight that summer. I stuck to LCHF/Keto religiously, but all I did was maintain.

105

I never felt like I had eaten a meal, and I was constantly hungry, so I ate and ate and ate. I think my body really prefers carbs for satiety, and eventually, my hair started falling out in a shocking way. I knew that it was time to reintroduce carbs, but I didn't want to regain the 25 pounds I had lost.

At that time, I remembered *The Carbohydrate Addict's Diet* (CAD) from the 1990s. I found a copy and started reading. If you think back to what I wrote about it in the chapter on adjusting to an intermittent fasting lifestyle, the premise of the CAD was that you ate two low carb meals during the day, and then you could have a reward meal of whatever you wanted, in an hour time frame. I started following the plan, and after that first meal with carbs, I felt immediately better. I actually started to lose weight slowly, even though I had added carbs back in to the nightly reward meal.

Summer was over, and it was time to go back to work. If you have ever eaten low carb, you know that it takes a lot of work to make sure you have the right foods with you. I had to pack a lunch and take it to school, and it had to be low carb. Ugh. I just couldn't do it. Too much work!

I thought about Rachael Heller's story. In the introduction to the CAD book, she explained how she discovered that she was a carbohydrate addict after she started skipping breakfast and lunch each day, and when she ate one meal per day, she had sanity around food for the first time in her life. (Sound familiar?) She lost a great deal of weight, and was able to maintain her loss over a long period of time. Of course, this was not the plan she promoted in her CAD book; I think the idea of not eating all day was too extreme, and she thought that people would be more open to a plan that allowed you to eat 3 meals per day.

I connected her original plan to what I remembered about Fast 5. Suddenly Fast 5 no longer sounded restrictive, as it had to me back in the 2009-2014 years. I had been living an extremely restrictive lifestyle for over three months, and the idea of a 5-hour eating window seemed positively luxurious. I immediately switched over to Fast 5, and my intermittent fasting lifestyle began in earnest.

I got the idea for daily weighing with weekly averaging from the CAD book, so I carried the habit into my intermittent fasting lifestyle. Finally, I had a consistent way to illustrate that I was losing weight every week, since my weekly average ALWAYS went down, even when my Friday-to-Friday weights were up slightly. I was so happy to finally be moving in the right direction again, even if it was very slow. Of course, this was the period where my goal was to maximize eating opportunities during the 5-hour window, and I was eating two meals every day. Even with the slow weight loss, I stuck with Fast 5 until October, when I "ran into" someone in the Fast 5 Facebook group who talked about a very fast weight loss plan called the 5 Bite Diet. (*Note: I would NEVER recommend this diet to anyone, now that I know better. NEVER. I am only including it here because I don't want to lie to you about how I lost my weight. I am very lucky that I didn't tank my metabolism, and I'm pretty sure that the only reason I didn't is because I lacked the willpower to continue longer than a few weeks. I know some wonderful ladies who had much more willpower than I did, and they followed this diet for a long period of time, perfectly, and they lost incredible amounts of weight. Do you know what else happened? They have had a terrible time maintaining their loss. They have to keep going back on the restrictive diet to keep their weight down, and it's all because they were MUCH more dedicated than I was. Don't do it. Don't try this diet. I beg you. In fact, don't try any of the crazy diets I did. Stick to intermittent fasting. Promise me.*)

Remember—I may have lost 35 pounds by this point, but I was still 40 pounds from my goal weight. I was still living with a diet mentality, and my only thought was to get to goal, and as fast as possible. I was ripe for a crash diet after losing at a snail's pace for so many months. How many of us fall for these crash diets and their promise of fast weight loss? DON'T DO IT, even if it is tempting.

The 5 Bite Diet (5BD) has a very interesting premise, and as familiar as I was with every diet ever written, it was a new one for me. It was written by a bariatric doctor who worked with patients who had weight loss surgery. He suggests that instead of having weight loss surgery, it makes a lot more sense to eat as if you had the surgery, but without mutilating your body. He recommends skipping breakfast, and then eating only 5 bites of food for lunch, and 5 bites of food for dinner. You don't have the surgery, but you eat as much food as if you had. 10 bites of food per day is not very much food. I started on October 29th of 2014 at 177 pounds, and after 7 days, I was already at 167.4. The weight loss was astonishing. Only hCG had previously allowed me to lose at this rate. After 14 days, I had gotten to 162.5, which was still 5 pounds in a week. One week later, I was down to 159.8. Suddenly, though, my weight seemed to plateau. Over the next 5 days, I didn't lose any weight at all. It was mid-November, and my body was SCREAMING at me to stop this crazy diet. Of course, it was—I was in danger of ruining my metabolism. Fortunately, I listened to my hormonal signals (remember—when you get an almost uncontrollable signal that you need to eat, it means you are doing something WRONG. You never want this feeling. It's an SOS from your body. Instead, what you want to feel is peace around food, while you slowly lose weight. Remember what I told you earlier about getting your hormones in balance.) I decided to go back to intermittent fasting to maintain the weight I lost on the 5 bite diet. It's no wonder that my body was mad at me--I calculated that I was only eating 500 calories or so per day, and I had done that for 25 days straight. Knowing what I know now, I'm not surprised that my weight loss stopped. I'm sure my metabolism was slowing down. As soon as I started back on intermittent fasting, my weight bounced back up to the lower 160s, and it stayed there until after Christmas.

Over that November/December season, I toyed around with several different intermittent fasting regimens. I tried Eat, Stop, Eat, which is one of the plans listed in the annotated bibliography. I would mix it up with days of Fast 5, and also I incorporated some up days/down days, in the style of alternate daily fasting. Overall, I managed to maintain a 12-pound loss from that round of the 5 bite diet by following various intermittent fasting techniques.

On December 28th of 2015, I realized I was ready to do another round of the 5BD. I was a glutton for punishment, and I apparently wanted more of it. The doctor who developed the diet suggested that you do it continually until you lose all of the weight you want to lose. I had 30 pounds to go to get to my goal weight, so I decided to commit. I weighed 165 pounds.

Fortunately, starving yourself is easier said than done. My body allowed me to stick with it for 21 days, and I lost 13 more pounds. However, I was miserable, the weight loss slowed to a crawl, and I instinctually knew this wasn't good for me. Again, I got all of the hormonal signals such as uncontrollable hunger, which should have alerted me that there was a problem. Keep in mind that this was before I learned about how long periods of calorie restriction slow the metabolism, and shows like the Biggest Loser were still teaching us that the faster you could lose the weight, the better. It was not the smartest thing I ever did. (DO NOT TRY IT!!!)

I did learn something interesting about myself during those 21 days, though. I learned that if I saved all 10 bites for dinner, it was easier. I could fast all day, and then eat a 500 calorie/10 bite dinner. I was eating one meal a day! It was so much easier than 2 smaller and less satisfying meals.

After abandoning the 5 bite diet for good (and I do mean FOREVER), I planned to go back to Fast 5, so I reread the Fast 5 book for inspiration. That's when I realized that Dr. Herring mentioned several times in his book that he was only eating one meal per day. Suddenly, it clicked: Fast 5 was initially intended to include one evening meal, not two shoved into a 5-hour period of time. I immediately began using a one meal a day (OMAD) approach. I weighed 152 pounds on January 20th, 2015, and I began OMAD in earnest. Because I wanted to lose weight faster, I limited myself to a window of about 1 hour most days, but I didn't count calories or restrict foods. I allowed myself to eat until I was satisfied every night. After all of the madness of the previous year, and all of the crazy restrictions, one meal a day felt luxurious. I reached 135 on March 17th, and declared myself officially at goal.

The one meal a day approach worked so much better than a 5-hour window had ever worked for me before. I was able to get to goal at the rate of about 2 pounds per week. That was much better than the pace of loss when I ate as much as I could in a 5-hour window.

I still wasn't convinced that OMAD was a lifestyle, but I knew that intermittent fasting WAS my ticket for long-term success. At that point, I was happily wearing a size 4 (and sometimes a 2!), and I understood that as long as I continued with intermittent fasting, and kept a close watch on my weight, I had the tools to keep the weight off forever. My confidence was high.

I maintained easily in the 130-132 range from March through the late fall of 2015. I experimented with several different intermittent fasting strategies during that time period. 5:2, with two full 36-42 hour fasts, suited me very well over the summer, and then when school started back, and I realized I was too lazy to pack a lunch for 3 of the 5 school days, I went back to eating one meal a day during the week. At that point, I got a bit cocky and decided that I should follow OMAD during the week and have "free weekends." This was in October of 2015. I slowly gained weight throughout November and December, and in January of 2016, I realized that I had gotten up to 138 pounds. If I continued to gain weight at that pace, I was afraid that I would be right back where I started from.

In January of 2016, I went back to one meal a day every day, but the weight didn't drop off this time. I managed to maintain in the mid to upper 130s, but I wanted to see the lower 130s again. I stuck with it, but the weight didn't budge. In late February, I decided that I needed to take more drastic measures, and I started doing 4:3, with 3 full fasts (36 hours) per week. Slowly, the weight started going down. I inched back down to the lower 130s.

Here is something to know about that time period in my life: I was using stevia constantly. I drank coffee all morning with stevia, and then I drank apple cinnamon flavored hot tea with more stevia all afternoon. I was constantly spiking my insulin, only I didn't realize what that was doing in my body.

In March, Dr. Fung's book, *The Obesity Code*, was released. I eagerly read it, cover to cover. He was insistent that we absolutely must stop using all sweeteners or sweet flavors during the fast, and that includes stevia. I kicked and screamed, but I did it. I drank my coffee black. I stopped drinking the sweet-flavored hot teas. I followed all fasting recommendations to keep insulin low during the fast.

The change was immediate. I lost more weight. The fast was easier. I didn't think so much about when it was time to eat. Could avoiding stevia and that sweet-flavored tea really have made such a difference for me? I think so, yes.

Right around that time, I realized that 4:3 was no longer easy. I dreaded the fasting days, and I even began to dread the up days, because I didn't like the way I felt when I ate 3 meals per day. I went back to my one meal a day lifestyle, and I've been doing it ever since.

I decided that I would limit myself to one meal a day, and I would focus on keeping my eating window to a time period of 5 hours or less. The switch from 4:3 to OMAD made me feel even better. Now that I had given up stevia, I finally understood appetite correction. I didn't think about food during the day, and my lifestyle was truly effortless. I knew that I had figured it out. I stopped spiking my insulin during the day, I ate according to my hunger signals each evening, and I felt better and better over time.

I stopped weighing myself in April of 2016, and haven't gotten on the scale since. I know that I have lost a few more pounds since then, but I am not really trying. I would estimate that my weight is in the upper 120s at this point, but I really don't care what the scale says. I went down one jeans size from May-September, and my fasting lifestyle feels truly effortless. This is what I do now. I eat one amazing meal every day, and if I need a snack before or after my meal, I have it. From May-early October I tracked my window length daily using an app my son made. I enjoyed tracking my window, and the app helped me be consistent. I learned that my average eating window is 2 1/2 hours per day, and that seems to be my sweet spot.

If you are interested in tracking your eating window, by the way, I highly recommend my son's app. The other apps tracked the length of the fast, and I wanted to track my eating window. Here is a link to his app in the Apple app store:
https://itunes.apple.com/us/app/window-intermittent-fasting/id1112765909?mt=8

It's called "Window Intermittent Fasting Tracker," by Cal Stephens, and it is only available for iPhone.

The way my day usually looks is this. I'll get home from work between 4:30-5:00 each day. Some days I choose to have a snack, and some days I don't. I may open my window at 4:30, or I might wait until 5:30. Other days, I wait even longer. Depending on my family's schedule, I usually

112

start cooking dinner somewhere between 5:00-6:00. If my window hasn't already opened before then, I will open it when cooking dinner. I taste things as I cook, and by the time dinner is done, I am ready for a great meal. We sit down for dinner, and I usually enjoy a glass of prosecco with my meal. After dinner, once the kitchen is cleaned up, I may decide that I want something sweet, and I'll eat a little something. Ice cream is one of my favorite treats, and I enjoy it often. As I mentioned before, nothing is off limits: I delay, and I don't deny!

On weekends, I often find myself watching the clock a bit more. Sometimes I'll open my window with a snack at 3:00, if I feel like I need one. My eating windows tend to be longer on Saturday and Sunday, but I still try to limit myself to no more than 5 hours. Some days, it's more like 6 hours, but usually, it is less than 5. One thing is for sure: I'm no longer having "free weekends," like I did back in the fall of 2015. I realized that doesn't work well for me. I feel better when keeping to a fasting schedule every day.

So—you've heard my whole crazy story. After all of my crazy attempts at dieting, for DECADES, I finally have peace and sanity. I am confident that I have found my permanent strategy. I am a little leaner today than I was last month. Eventually, I figure my body will settle at whatever is my "ideal" weight, but I'm not focused on the numbers anymore.

As I continue fasting, I am noticing that any loose or wrinkly skin that I have is tightening up. My arms look toned, even though I don't work out. My belly looks better than it used to, even though I know I'll never have a fitness model belly. (I am 47 years old, had two babies, and I used to weigh 210 pounds. No way is that belly going to ever be perfect, and that is okay.)

The longer I fast, the better my body shape becomes. Thanks, autophagy! I have more energy than I have ever had in my life. I look younger now than I did ten years ago.

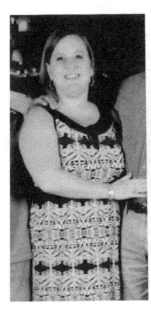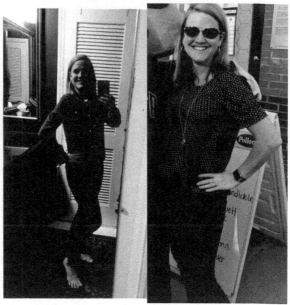

The first picture is from April of 2014, when I weighed 210 pounds. The second is in the spring of 2015, when I weighed between 130-135. The third is one year after I reached goal, in the spring of 2016. I am wearing the same pants in the 2nd and 3rd photos. Since the 3rd photo was taken, I have gotten a little leaner as the months have gone by. Intermittent fasting: THANK YOU!

Appendix B: 30 journal prompts

Face it—so much of the weight loss process is mental, and we would all agree that there is a huge emotional component surrounding food. We celebrate with food; we reward ourselves with food—in fact, it's impossible to avoid delicious food.

Journaling is a powerful process. I haven't officially journaled in a notebook, but I have written many Facebook posts in the many weight loss groups I've been a member of over the years. Writing out my thoughts and feelings has been so very helpful to me. Basically, I have made the whole world my weight loss journal. You may not want to be as public about your struggles as I have been, so a private journal just for you may be more to your liking.

I have given you 30 journal prompts here. Buy yourself a small notebook, set up a document on your computer or your tablet, or just staple a few sheets of paper together, and begin a journal. The purpose is to really think about why you eat, and how food makes you feel. You can use these prompts one by one in order, you can skip around and write about the ones that speak directly to you on any given day, or you can deviate from these prompts entirely and write whatever helps you personally.

After you have exhausted these prompts, continue your journaling by writing about any successes, failures, or revelations you experience. Or, you could be like me, and join some Facebook groups or other internet support forums and interact with others there. No matter what format you decide on, there is something powerful about writing down your thoughts.

1: What does food mean to me?

2: "I deserve to be slim and vibrant more than I deserve to eat recreationally." How does that thought make me feel?

3: What lies do I tell myself about food and eating?

4: Why do I eat/want to eat more than my body needs?

5: How will I handle naysayers who say that fasting is bad for me?

6: How important is the scale to me? What if I don't see quick progress? How will I cope with that?

7: When I am bored, and want to eat, what can I do instead?

8: Why do I want to lose weight? Really—deep down—WHY?

9: Other than food, how can I reward myself?

10: Do I ever keep eating when I am full? If so, why do I do that, and how can I stop?

11: How will I handle social situations where I feel pressured to eat, but I don't want to eat?

12: What foods make me feel good, and what foods make me feel bad?

13: How will my life change if I can get control of my eating/my weight?

14: What has stopped me from losing weight in the past?

15: How do I define success when it comes to this lifestyle?

16: What behavioral goals can I set for myself? (*Note: behavioral goals are more powerful than "pounds to lose" goals. This is because you can control your behavior, but you can't control how much weight your body releases in a given time period.*)

17: What habits support my weight loss/health goals? What habits work against me?

18: Who can support me as I work through this process? Friends? Family? A partner?

19: How do I feel about the thought that this lifestyle is FOREVER? That this isn't a plan you stop when you get to "goal"?

20: What, besides eating, brings me JOY?

21: How do I feel during the day when I fast? How does that compare to days when I don't fast?

22: How do my clothes feel on my body? Are they getting looser or tighter?

23: How do I make a switch from "diet" mentality to "lifestyle" mentality? Do I need to?

24: When did I feel best in my body? How old was I? How did I eat at that time? Can I learn any lessons from that version of me?

25: What does "delay, don't deny" mean to me?

26: How do I define a special occasion, when it is okay to feast rather than fast?

27: Do I have some foods that I consider to be "good" foods and some that I consider to be "bad" foods? How can I break free of the labels I have given to food, so that food doesn't have as much power over me?

28: How do I want to teach the next generation (my kids, my grandkids) to approach food and eating? What lessons do I want to pass down?

29: When I reflect upon my own history related to foods and diets, what lessons have I learned about myself?

30: How does it feel to finally have control of my eating behaviors?

Appendix C: Annotated Bibliography

All of these outstanding books are available from any of your favorite online book retailers. Every single one of them was instrumental in shaping my understanding of how the body works. Any errors I have made in the summaries about the content of the books are mine, and mine alone. I would recommend any of them, and I would love for you to support these pioneering authors by purchasing their books.

These books aren't listed alphabetically, in order of publication, or according to any other accepted form of bibliography formatting. Instead, I have arranged the books in order on a scale from "completely changed my life" to "also a great resource." I also haven't given you publisher names, copyright dates, ISBN numbers, or any sort of formal information. I am assuming you know how to go to your favorite book seller's website and search by book title. That will get you to each one of these books. Happy reading!

The Fast-5 Diet, **by Dr. Bert Herring** Of course, I have to list this book first. If you have read my story, you know that the Fast 5 plan was my introduction to intermittent fasting, and I first read this book in 2009 or so. Even though it took me YEARS to finally commit, I kept returning to this plan until it finally clicked for me. Dr. Herring writes this book in a very approachable way, and it's an easy plan to follow. If you read it, look for his casual comments about eating "one meal" every day, and understand that you probably aren't going to be very successful if your goal is to eat as much as you can in a 5-hour period.

Dr. Herring is a true pioneer in the intermittent fasting community, and I am eternally grateful to him for his work. (One caveat: after reading *The Obesity Code*, I no longer agree with his recommendations about drinking diet sodas while fasting. He takes more of a "try it and see if it works for you" approach, while I am hardcore "DON'T DO IT...INSULIN RELEASE!!!!" If you read *The Obesity Code*, you will be the same way.) Dr. Herring also has a website and provides health coaching for a fee. If you need more personalized support than a Facebook group could give you, check out his health coaching services.

The Obesity Code, **by Dr. Jason Fung** This book changed my life even though it was not the first book I read on fasting, and I had already reached my goal weight before I read it. This was the one that really helped me understand how the body works—it tied together all of the loose ends that I picked up along the way, into one cohesive big picture. It was after reading this book that I accepted the fact that I needed to give up my beloved stevia during my fast. BOY, was that hard, but the science he outlines is so compelling. Anyone who reads this and then decides to continue using any sort of insulin-stimulating products during the fast—I just don't get it. I had so many "a-ha" moments while reading this book! One thing to know about it: it is not always an easy read. It is long. You may need to re-read sections to understand the science. If you are impatient and want something that is quick and to the point, you may not enjoy this book. I, however, have read it multiple times, and every time I do, I learn something new about the body. Dr. Fung explains how important hormones, specifically insulin, are the key to the weight loss process. He also discusses the many benefits of fasting, and how what you eat can make a difference. I do think that he could have been more specific about how to fast, and apparently, he agreed with me, because within a year, he released a second book called *The Complete Guide to Fasting*. The second book is further down on my list, because it didn't teach me anything I didn't already know. That being said, it may be a better choice for anyone who is looking for a less science-y book.

AC: The Power of Appetite Correction, **by Dr. Bert Herring**
Yes, Dr. Herring is on my list twice. This book was released when I was part-way through my weight loss journey, and it gave me one HUGE "a-ha" moment that has had a permanent impact on my mindset. I'm not sure that I would be where I am today without having made that mental shift. In this book, he introduces us to the concept of "appetite correction" (AC), and I think it is genius. He really makes it clear that while intermittent fasting, we need to keep modifying what we are doing until we reach the holy land of AC. The thing about appetite correction: you know it when you feel it. Suddenly, fasting isn't a struggle. You stop eating when you are full. Everything clicks into place when you reach AC! He's absolutely right, and understanding the power of AC helped me realize how I personally needed to approach intermittent fasting. I didn't have AC when I used stevia during the fast. I didn't have AC when I did 4:3. I didn't have AC when I tried to cram two meals into a 5-hour window. I don't even have great AC when I open my window a little earlier, at 3 p.m. Over time, and with lots of trial and error, I understand that I have the best AC when I wait until 5 pm to open my window. When I do that, I don't have to time myself while I eat or consciously restrict. This is the goal that every one of us is looking for: you want to be in a place where you are listening to satiety signals, and you are not fasting through sheer willpower alone. When you understand AC, you can experiment until you get there.

The Science of Skinny, **by Dee McCaffrey** I don't even
follow Dee's recommendations for what to eat, but I
still have this book up high on my list, because it's a
great introduction to what we should eat and what
we shouldn't eat (in theory). I did follow her
suggestions briefly (very briefly) along the way, but it
was just too hard for me to commit to processed-free
living. I did realize, however, that I feel REALLY
GOOD when the bulk of my diet is made up of real
food, as in what our great-great-grandparents ate.
That realization affects my choices to this day,
because I would rather feel good than eat total crap.
I'm certain I would be healthier and leaner if I stuck
to her guidelines, but I just don't want to, darn it. If
you read this book, overlook her recommendations
about eating frequent meals; we are intermittent
fasters, after all. I'm certain Dee would be very upset
with me if she met me. She is completely anti-sugar,
and I eat sugar every day; she doesn't like refined
grains, and I eat them every day; she wants you to eat
frequently, and I fast every day…you get it. I don't
follow her recommendations. Sigh. That being said,
if I started gaining weight, or wanted to lose more
weight and was having trouble, I would not hesitate
to tweak my diet to include more of her guidelines. I
believe she lays out a sensible plan for how to eat for
health, but I just like processed food too much. Bread.
Ice cream. Cookies. Yes, yes, and yes. I am happily
delaying, rather than denying; though I do sometimes
think about her recommendations when I am
deciding between two things—all other factors being
equal, I'll select the lesser-processed item in her
honor. Also, thanks to this book, I am more likely to
incorporate nutritious foods into my eating window.
I eat a lot more veggies than I used to, for example.

The Carbohydrate Addict's Diet, **by Drs. Richard and
Rachael Heller** Again, here is another plan that I
don't follow, but it is high on my list because it
helped steer me towards the one meal a day lifestyle.

122

It's not even available in e-format, and you want the old version from 1991, which you'll probably have to buy as a used paperback. The pure gold is in the introduction, where Rachael describes her weight loss struggles and eventual epiphany. She was finally able to lose weight when she started skipping breakfast and lunch and only eating dinner, all thanks to a rescheduled doctor's appointment that required her to be in the fasted state. Rachael invented intermittent fasting and discovered appetite correction, but she didn't even know it. She reached the nirvana of appetite correction by eating one meal a day for dinner, went on to lose all of her weight, and maintained effortlessly. Sound familiar? If not, reread my chapter on the one meal a day lifestyle. She was living it before it was a thing. The actual plan listed in the book is a combination of low carb meals with one daily reward meal, at which time you can eat whatever you want within a one-hour eating window. This book was truly before its time, as the principles make complete sense when you view her recommendations through the lens of *The Obesity Code*. I believe that intermittent fasting with one meal per day, which is what she actually DID, is more powerful than the low carb plan she recommends; however, if you are having trouble adjusting to an intermittent fasting lifestyle, I would 100% recommend that you start with her book's plan and work your way up to the one meal plan.

The Complete Guide to Fasting, **by Dr. Jason Fung and Jimmy Moore** I already mentioned this book in the section for *The Obesity Code*, and I told you that it is listed farther down my list because I didn't learn anything new. I was so excited for this book to be released, and was a bit disappointed when it actually came out. Still, it is a good choice if you find *The Obesity Code* to be too tedious for you. I want to warn you: because Jimmy is a co-author, this book has a decidedly LCHF/Keto slant. Heck, even Dr. Fung has that LCHF/Keto slant in many of his blog posts. If you know Jimmy Moore, you'll recognize him from the low carb community, and you also know that he has written several books related to following a LCHF/Keto lifestyle. Since Dr. Fung promotes insulin control as the key to managing weight (and health), it was only natural that the LCHF/Keto community would embrace his work. This book is an example of the collaboration between the two. Before reading this book, you need to understand something about Jimmy Moore: even though he follows LCHF/Keto, he has had a hard time maintaining his weight loss, and also never reached his final goal weight. Thanks to his collaboration with Dr. Fung, he is using fasting—both long fasts and intermittent fasts—to help him make more progress. Even though I personally delay, rather than deny, I recognize that there are people who are so insulin resistant that they may need to incorporate LCHF/Keto strategies, along with intermittent fasting, to truly reach their goals. This book is a great resource for anyone looking to combine the two approaches. Which is not going to be me. Nope. #ILoveYouCarbs

Good Calories, Bad Calories, **by Gary Taubes** I LOVED this book when it came out in 2008. It's nonfiction, but it reads like a thriller in certain sections. Taubes weaves his way through years—decades—CENTURIES, even—of nutrition dogma, and shoots holes in many commonly held theories. High cholesterol is bad? IS IT? Is it REALLY? He questions everything we have been told, and when I read this book, I realized that not all beliefs we hold as true are based on solid scientific studies. Just like Dr. Fung, Taubes questions the legitimacy of the calories in/calories out (CI/CO) theory, and ever since I read this book, I haven't believed that CI/CO is either as simple as most people think, or as accurate. As Dr. Fung does in *The Obesity Code,* Taubes makes a case for insulin being the driver of obesity, rather than calories. Once you understand that, you understand why fasting works so well for weight loss (especially when you take great care to prevent insulin spikes during your fast, as I recommend). I haven't read this book in years, but once I get my book published (and if you are reading it, you'll see I did!), and I have some time on my hands again, I think I will give it a good re-read.

Why We Get Fat and What to do About It, by Gary Taubes This was his follow up to *Good Calories, Bad Calories*. As in the first book, Taubes discusses how many of the commonly held beliefs about diet and nutrition are flat-out wrong. CI/CO—completely destroyed. Once again, Taubes makes a case for insulin being the driver of obesity, rather than calories. When this book came out, I gave LCHF one more try, and it STILL didn't work for me. As I mentioned in earlier sections of the book, I don't feel well when I follow a LCHF lifestyle, and I also love carbs. I can't stick to LCHF, and even when I did make myself stick to it for a couple of months, I didn't lose any weight. I just can't lose weight when I eat all day, no matter what I am eating. No, for me, I don't lower my insulin by eating LCHF all day long, I lower it by using intermittent fasting. The underlying science, however, is the same. If you understand the principles in this book, you understand why intermittent fasting works so well, thanks to the insulin control it provides. I am going to re-read this book, right after I re-read *Good Calories, Bad Calories*. Both are excellent. By the way, Gary Taubes has a new release called *The Case Against Sugar*, and I am not even going to look directly at it in the Kindle store, because I am not about to give up sugar. I'll give it up for 19-23 hours of every day, since I am fasting, but that is IT. Sorry, Gary. No.

The Every Other Day Diet, by Dr. Krista Varady This is an excellent book, and I highly recommend it to anyone considering an alternate day fasting (ADF) approach.

Dr. Varady has done a great deal of research in a university setting on ADF, and she has reported great results from the strategy. She suggests that you eat a 400-calorie lunch or dinner plus a 100-calorie snack on the down days, which she calls diet days. Personally, I found that I was able to comply with the diet days better when my calorie intake was 0, because once I start eating, it is hard for me to stop. She also recommends lunch specifically for your 400 calorie meal, and I know myself—if I tried to eat a 400 calorie lunch and then eat nothing else (besides a 100 calorie snack) I would be so hangry that everyone would have to avoid me for the rest of the day. It is SO MUCH EASIER for me to eat nothing at all than it is to stick to a tiny meal. You may find that you do very well with a 500-calorie day, however. If you want to try ADF, this is the book I would recommend first.

The Alternate-Day Diet, **by Dr. James Johnson** I read this book before I read *The Every Other Day Diet*, but I like Varady's book a little better because of her research. Still, this is another great ADF plan. His plan is often referred to in diet circles as the "JUDDD" plan, which stands for "Johnson's Up Day/Down Day" plan. I am pretty sure that he is the person who came up with the "up day" "down day" terms.

The Fast Diet, **by Michael Mosley and Mimi Spencer** I really wanted this plan to work for me, because it is so easy: pick any 2 days per week, and fast, and the rest of the time, eat normally. It's what we call 5:2. In this plan, as with the ADF plans, fast days are really 500 calorie days, and you can spread them out throughout the day however you want. I used my own version of 5:2 for maintenance, and rather than eating 500 calories on the 2 down days, I did full fasts and went to bed without having eaten anything. 5:2 is just not enough fasting for me to lose weight, though thousands of people have success with it.

The 5:2 Diet, **by Kate Harrison** Kate Harrison takes the plan developed by Michael Mosley, which was originally not a book, and puts it into book form. Confused? Let me explain. Dr. Mosley first presented his work in a BBC documentary (*Horizon: Eat, Fast, and Live Longer*), where the concept of 5:2 was actually born. Kate Harrison took the ideas from the documentary and put them into this book. Later, Dr. Mosley and Mimi Spencer wrote their own book. Whichever plan came first, they are both the same: 2 days of 500-calorie "fast" days, and 5 days of "eating normally."

Eat, Stop, Eat, **by Brad Pilon** This book was initially sold through Brad Pilon's website at www.eatstopeat.com. Brad is an internet marketer, so you'll see all sorts of hype on his website prompting you to BUY NOW! to unlock the secrets of intermittent fasting! Even if you don't buy it, it's worth a trip to his website to take a look at him, because he is a bodybuilder and is ripped. Even though a muscle-bound man isn't my preference (my husband is lanky), Brad does have a gorgeous physique, and there is no harm in a quick peek. Go ahead. I'll wait… Brad illustrates through his own physique that fasting is NOT going to cause you to lose muscle mass like many critics claim. Brad's actual plan involves a couple of 24-hour fasts every week, which you do as a dinner-to-dinner fast. It works well for him (a bodybuilder with LOADS of muscle mass and very little fat), but it is definitely not enough fasting for me to lose weight. Still, it's a great illustration of the concept that fasting won't destroy your muscle mass (and I do mean a GREAT illustration).

The Warrior Diet, **by Ori Hofmekler** This is such an interesting book, even though it is pretty far down on my list. Ori Hofmekler presents a case for eating like a warrior: fast during the day, and then feast at night. Actually, he calls the part during the day the "undereating" phase, so you aren't really fasting in the way we understand it. It's ALMOST intermittent fasting, but not quite, because he allows you to eat small amounts of things during the day, such as fruit. He provides some interesting historical context to the idea of feasting every night, which is why I included this book on my list. I wouldn't recommend following it the way he has it written, because you aren't really fasting; instead, read it for the historical insight, but follow it using the fasting recommendations I give in this book during the day. If you do, you are following the one meal a day plan, which you know is my favorite, and the way I am currently living my life.

The Calorie Myth, **by Jonathan Bailor** This book is pretty far down on my list, but it was another that shaped my current thinking about calories. Just as Dr. Fung, Gary Taubes, and Dee McCaffrey insist, Jonathan Bailor explains that all calories are not equal within the body. I like any book that shoots holes in the calories in/calories out myth, which is why I included this one. Honestly—in my opinion, anyone who still believes that all calories are treated the same in the body just hasn't read very much about nutrition. While we all know that you could lose weight eating nothing but twinkies, we also understand that you aren't going to get the same results if you eat 2000 calories of twinkies each day vs. 2000 calories of raw vegetables. Also, you are going to have terrible long-term results on this type of twinkie-plan. If you still don't believe it, either conduct a study of one (using yourself) or read this book.

Appendix D: Testimonials: Fasting WORKS!

In my years of intermittent fasting, I have met some truly inspiring people who have used intermittent fasting to get their health back. Here are some of their stories. In their own words, they will tell you how intermittent fasting has changed their lives. I have to admit—this is my favorite part of the whole book.

You don't have to take it from me: intermittent fasting not only works, it changes lives. Notice the common thread in these stories: just like me, most of these people have tried diet after diet over the years, and many had given up on ever being slim—until they discovered intermittent fasting.

Enjoy these inspiring stories of success and hope!

Shirley Jean:
BREAKING FREE FROM DIETS!!!

I have been a yo-yo dieter for about 45 years. I have been on just about every diet you can think of with my lowest weight just under 130 and my highest at 230. I have literally spent thousands on commercial programs, pills, powders, shakes, diet books, gym memberships, exercise equipment, exercise books, & videos. I even worked for one year as a weight loss counselor for a well-known commercial weight-loss center, believing I could finally lose my weight and learn from "the experts" how to keep it off!! Ironically, I was chosen to also lead the "Lifestyle" classes. So much for learning from "the experts." I did lose 28 pounds, but eventually became tired of the same old food, most of it not filling, satisfying, nor tasty. Whenever I embarked on my newest endeavor to drop weight, I found myself with a completely focused mindset, determined that THIS time, I was going to reach my coveted goal weight number and magically, I would maintain that number!! Alas, the few times I met that goal, I remained there for a very, very brief time. I just wasn't willing to continue with those diet foods, powders, shakes, pills, and endless meetings for the rest of my life!! Since I never learned how to maintain my new size, I always had anxiety about keeping my weight off. The lost weight would creep back on until I started the next diet. Vicious cycle. About 2-3 years ago, I started hearing about IF, and after trying various IF protocols, I heard about Gin's One Meal a Day (OMAD) Facebook group. I was intrigued because I had done this before with great success. Back in the late 70s, I read a book with a crazy title: "The EATFYL diet," which stood for "eat all the foods you love" in one hour, once per day. I did this, enjoyed it, and was very successful losing the 15 pounds I wanted to lose. I viewed this "diet" as a temporary means to lose my excess fat, never as a maintenance plan. Without the research to back it up and no support group like we have today, I did gain back the weight. After a few brief attempts with OMAD over the past year or so, I became serious about OMAD with Gin's September 2016 challenge on her Facebook group. I started out in my typical way, in a rush to get to my goal weight. I projected into the future with a laid out plan...if I lose X amount of weight each week, then I will reach X weight by X date. I weighed myself frequently and charted my weight on a graph. I also weighed and measured my food, kept a food journal, and counted calories. Thanks to Gin and her no-weighing philosophy, I eventually realized that the scale has never helped me to succeed. It's always been a love-hate relationship and quite a roller coaster ride. In early November, I decided to stop weighing for a while, which meant I stopped charting my weight on a graph. It also meant I would stop projecting my weight loss into the future. Wow...that's three "diet behaviors"!!! I then decided to examine other "diet behaviors" of mine, such as keeping a food journal, counting calories, and weighing and measuring my food. I had an epiphany as I realized that all this weighing and measuring and counting and tracking of my body and my food reinforced in my mind that OMAD was just another diet and not a permanent lifestyle...for me. I made the decision to stop any behaviors that felt like diet behaviors to me. I no longer track anything, and I no longer focus on numbers.

My focus is to continue OMAD each day, one day at a time, knowing I'm continuing to get smaller. I'm not 100% perfect on this journey, but I AM making progress. When I last weighed myself in early November, I was down about 42 pounds from my highest weight, with 23 pounds of that lost with OMAD since August 31, 2016. I do want to release more weight, but I have no "goal weight" number. Right now, my goal is not a number. My goal is FREEDOM to enjoy food, without guilt, without deprivation, without weighing and measuring and counting and tracking. And I'm there!!! I'm living AT MY GOAL! THIS is my permanent lifestyle. THIS is my "maintenance"!!!

Robin:

I finally did it! It took eight years, but I've now lost 100 pounds! I'm just 5 pounds from a 'normal' BMI. I can't thank Dr. Jason Fung enough for giving me the info I needed to make it happen. I believe Gin was the one who first posted his YouTube series for me to see. That series changed my life. I surely could have done things faster had I had his info earlier. Keto + fasting = what works for me.

I've done a little bit of everything as I think it's good to switch things up. When I first started, eating one meal a day didn't allow me to lose. So I did longer, 42-hour fasts maybe 3x per week. Then I added LCHF/Keto, and that helped, too. I also sometimes do multi-day fasts where the first two days are a fat fast, and then the next 1-2 days are just coffee with a little cream. I think changing things helps. Now I can still continue to lose with two keto meals a day, but I'll continue to work longer fasts in as I try to lose maybe 10-15 more pounds.

K. S.:

I have been eating one meal a day (dinner) for almost 20 years. I had no idea that this was a "thing." In fact, I have been fairly secretive about it due to people's reactions and in order to avoid being accused of having an eating disorder. Whenever I am confronted by people from work or family about my eating habits, I usually act casual and change the subject because nobody really understands how well this has worked for me. I started by accident in 1998 when I was 20 years old and worked as a waitress. I would start work at 6:00 p.m. and have dinner at work. Then I would work all night, get home at 2 or 3 a.m., go to sleep, wake up in the afternoon, and go to work. This is how my one meal a day journey started. My body adjusted quickly and kept this up after leaving my waitressing job and going back to school. Within a year, I had lost about 50 lbs. I kept the weight off for many years. In 2011, I gained a few pounds, probably because of age, but was still well within a normal weight. Now two babies later...lost most of that baby weight (although blew up in both pregnancies). I'm not as strict as I used to be but still maintain my one meal a day diet on most days. I literally can't function if I eat lunch now. I'm just way too tired. Anyway, that's my story.

Amanda:

I've always been a chubby person. I remember weighing 150 pounds in the 5th grade. When I was 18, I started skipping breakfast and lunch and just ate dinner. At the time I was unaware of fasting, and was just tired of being overweight. I don't know what I started at then, probably 165 pounds or so, but standing at 5'6". I got down to 140 pounds, size 4 jeans. Then my fiancé came along. I got a little comfortable, gained some. Then after we married, I packed on the pounds and was up to 185 pounds, which at the time I remember it being the biggest I had ever been. I got tired of it and started dieting again. I've never much been a breakfast person, so I just started skipping lunch, which left dinner. And I walked like a crazy person! I would get up every day and walk 2-3 miles before work at 1 p.m. in the afternoon in the hot summer, and then at work, I was walking non-stop for 10 hours straight, and I purposely would go up and down stairs more than needed. I never used my step counter at work, but trust me, it was a lot! I got back down to 140 pounds again. That's my ideal weight. Again, at the time I had never heard of fasting or anything, so I didn't tell anyone, and I would still drink sugary stuff, so it wasn't a true fast, but I was only eating once a day, and it's part of my journey.

After that came two kids. After the first baby, I weighed 165 pounds and kept that for several years. We tried several times to have a second baby, and we lost two in the process. I was depressed and gave up hope. Food was my friend. When I got pregnant again with my daughter, I was up to 190 pounds. I'm hypoglycemic, and when I was pregnant with her, it was crazy how fast and hard an episode would hit me. I took a nap once and woke up having a bad episode and remember scooting down the stairs on my butt because I was too weak to walk and I had to keep stopping and forcing myself to stay awake because I kept going in and out, and then I crawled to the kitchen and grabbed a box of cereal and laid on the kitchen floor eating as fast as I could, hoping I could stop it before passing out. It was the worst episode I've ever had, and it was scary as hell. After that, I remember making sure to eat every hour. A sandwich, an apple, a cookie, it didn't matter, just something to keep my sugar from plummeting. My husband works a lot, and I had a toddler to care for. I couldn't risk being home by myself with him and having another bad episode. He

133

wasn't even old enough to understand 9-1-1. So, after I had her, I weighed 203 pounds.

After a few years of focusing on taking care of the kids and ignoring myself, I weighed 216 pounds at my heaviest. It was the summer of 2014. We took the kids to a theme park, and my husband took a picture of me on a ride with the kids. When I saw the picture, I was horrified, disgusted, and tired of being overweight. I started skipping meals again and started riding my bike every night. By Christmas that year I was down to 178! I felt good, and I stopped trying. Then, in April of 2015, when I realized I had gained and was back up to 185, I was upset. That's when I got really serious. I went back to just eating dinner, but at that time I had joined a fasting group who thinks it's only about calories in/calories out (CI/CO), and I didn't know any better at the time, so I was still having my coffee with sugar and cream in the morning, would eat dinner, and then go for a run. After that, I'd drink some wine. I also started doing Jillian Michael's 30-day shred workout every morning. I worked up to running 6 miles every night. By August, I was down to 143 pounds! I felt great, full of energy, and I was happy with myself and life again. I could cross my legs again. I could see my collar bones again. I could run miles upon miles without stopping. I could go outside and play with my kids without tiring out. I wore size-2 jeans for the first time in my life!!

I maintained that through spring of this year and it had crept back up to 156 pounds. But once I joined the OMAD Facebook group and have started fasting the correct way, I've lost 3 pounds. I love fasting the correct way. I'm NOT hungry, and I eat less during my meal times, whereas before when I was having sugar/cream coffee in the morning, I was miserable all day until dinner. I've been sick nonstop for the past 2 months and being on medicines that require to be taken with food morning and night, I've not been able to really jump in, but the few times I've been off meds I've been successful, lost the 3 pounds, and have kept myself from creeping up higher. I just started a new medicine Friday that's got to be taken for 14 days, so I'm going to watch how much I eat and try to still fast for 16 hours so that I'm doing some fasting, but still taking my medicine with a little food so I don't get sick.

Here's a picture of me at my heaviest and in the spring when I was down to my ideal weight. I started at 216 pounds, size 16/18 jeans, and got to 143 pounds and could comfortably wear a 4, and sometimes a 2, depending on the brand. With OMAD, I will get back to my ideal weight again. I have before, and I'll do it again, but this time I will do it the right way, and I'll maintain this way of eating. It really is the best!

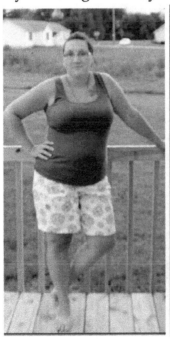 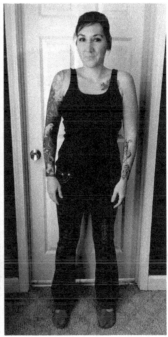

Hanaa:

I am Hanaa from Egypt. I am 53, but I was only 29 after having my first child back in 1992 when I had to travel to France with my husband for two years. I was 58 kg, only 3 kilos above my pre-pregnancy weight and quite satisfied. In France, everything changed. The media to the petite French women preached a svelte physique. I got the feeling I was fat, and started counting calories every day, exceeding my limit, failing, blowing it and bingeing to start over the next day. And my bulimia started too, with depression.

I came back to Egypt 60 plus kg, depressed, bulimic and perpetually dieting. They started me on antidepressants, and I became really fat. Between 1994 and 2012 I went from 62 to 90 kg. And all through those years, there wasn't a day I wasn't dieting! I tried several times to get off the antidepressants but relapsed every time, so I'm on them for life now. I did manage to lose around 12 kilos several times during those years with dietician's help only to gain them with a few extra kilos each time. I lost money on dieticians, diet books, health foods, diet medicines…etc. I developed cancer of the breast in 2012 and thought I'd lose weight with the chemotherapy but didn't. But I realized I was killing myself.

One day I was browsing Amazon for yet another diet book when they suggested I purchase Dr. Moseley's *Fast Diet* book. I clicked only because I thought "fast" meant "quick." Fasting was the last thing on my mind: I was unable to fast even for religious causes. But I was so desperate I ordered the book.

I started on 5-2 fasting in 2013 because I thought if I could eat without restriction in quantity or quality for 5 days, it was worth restricting for 2 non-consecutive days. With time my appetite got tamed. It took almost 1 year to lose 10 kilos. Then I became impatient and wanted quicker results. I spent 2014 and a good part of 2015 doing the five bite diet and completely failing. But I never regained those 10 kilos. I think it was because there is some sort of fasting involved in five bite, and I was hooked on fasting. I just can't take any food before 4 p.m. now.

In September 2015 I started on *The Every Other Day Diet* after reading the book. By December I had lost another 10 kilos. After that, the 36-hour fasts seemed unsustainable, and I've been on Dr. Bert Herring's Fast Five diet ever since. I don't lose on it because the eating window is too long, I think, and I eat too much. I found Gin's wonderful group and started seriously on OMAD (one meal a day), hoping to lose the last 10 plus kilos. I'm not in a hurry. I'm working on myself to stop or limit added sugars during regular days (not all carbs). And to incorporate some sort of extended fast once every month.

Besides the weight loss my HbA1c has gone from 6 to 4.8, and last time I had my abdominal sonar, the physician found no evidence of the non-alcoholic fatty liver I used to have.

Brian Siemon:

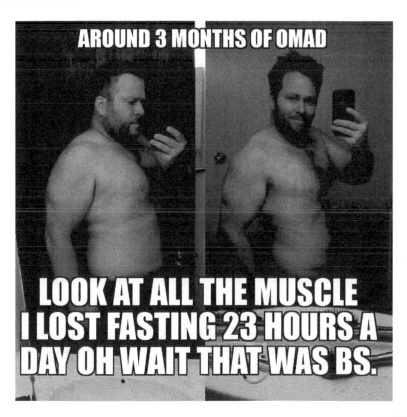

Somewhere in the 2000s I was in California and had gained weight to 280 pounds. I have never been super small. I weighed 180 in high school and was in pretty good shape. I started working out and eating better. I was able to lose 30 pounds, then moved back to Spokane and joined a gym. I worked hard to diet and work out to 195 from 250. I did a lot of cardio at the time, so I had lost 85 pounds, but hadn't gotten to see my abs. I moved away from my gym and stopped working out, started dating a girl as well, and eventually gained back to 271 when I got married. We went on Weight Watchers free-style, counting points or whatever. Lost a bit; I think 20. We stopped doing that, and we both gained weight. I think I was still around 270ish and we did hCG and lost down to 220 lbs. As soon as we stopped starving ourselves, we gained the weight all back. I hovered at 280. Next, I tried vegan for 6 months.

Then I lost my wife in 2014. I didn't weigh myself, but had the crazy idea that no way was I over 300 pounds. Then one day I stood on the scale at my in-laws and saw I was at 328 pounds. I didn't weigh again, so I could have been over 330 when I started working out. The first thing I did was get my gym membership back and started going to the gym. I cut my eating and started counting calories and doing about an hour of cardio and then one hour of weights 5 days a week. Sometimes more.

I ate lots of veggies and would end up skipping breakfast sometimes because it felt better to work out on just coffee even though I added caramel creamer. I did that low-calorie diet for 6 months and was able to get down under 300 pounds. I felt a lot better even though I was still heavy.

In August I stumbled upon intermittent fasting. I think after one day I had just drunk coffee, worked out, and then didn't eat all day. I remember feeling that I should eat and I could eat, but I wasn't really in need of food.

I found the Warrior Diet, which is fruits and nuts during the day and a feast at night. I discovered the words "intermittent fasting" and looked up a ton. I watched a ton of videos and read a bunch of studies. Some were bogus, and some were just about fasting. I read some blogs about fasting and saw results. The biggest thing I noticed was a lot of the blogs or stories ended with "and all this can be yours for $39.99."

So the next day I stopped eating during the day and had just one meal at night. I read all about hunger hormones among a hundred other new vocabulary words. I non-stop Googled. I drank my black coffee, drank a ton of water, and ate one meal. I have deviated on three occasions. Two were vacations, two days each, and I longed to go back to one meal. My body craves it. The other was a Tres Leche cake I needed to try, so I did. Even though I think it triggered some hunger I was in the life and knew the real hunger vs. the hormonal hunger. I haven't reached my goal yet, which is to be ripped. But this is the easiest way to lose weight. I don't restrict anything although I don't eat some things I used to since it's just not worth it to my taste buds.

My total weight today is 76 pounds lost. My average weight loss from March is about 1.97 pounds a week. That average keeps going up since I have lost way more in the last three months vs. the first six months of following Calories in/Calories Out (CICO).

Bev:

This is the short version of my story. I weighed around 300 pounds in the 1980s. I was depressed, and I prayed to the Lord, and He led me to eating only one meal per day and walking. It took me two years to lose 150 pounds. I ate one meal, with no more than 870 calories per meal. I started out eating frozen dinners because I could not cook. I had been on every diet known to man. All of my life. At an early age, I took diet pills – black beauties, and others. The most I had lost before trying one meal a day was 70 pounds – and I gained it back. With the one meal, I was successful. Mostly because I believe in obedience to the Lord. Obedience paid off and royally.

Through that journey, like I said, I started with frozen dinners, and I rewarded myself with something sweet. The downside to this was the bondage of counting calories. During my journey, I also stopped eating meat (I am back to eating meat now). For a decade, I ate vegetarian. That was extremely difficult. Back then it was difficult where I lived to eat that way. You had to be creative. I ate a lot of beans. I joined the Facebook group because I wanted the fellowship with others that are doing it also. I am just doing what I did back in the late 80's early 90's. I had never heard of Dr. Fung. I like the way that I do it because it is proven successful for me. I no longer count calories. Most times I eat at 1 p.m., and I stop when I am full. I don't eat any more until the next day. If I eat any later, like 5 p.m. – I am preoccupied with food the entire night. Getting enough calories is not an issue, because I eat lavishly…good fat, good meat, and good sweets (sometimes – I am getting to where at the end of the meal, I have no room for the sweets. I allow my body to dictate).

Robin Lopez, from Modesto, CA:
  Here's my story. When I was in high school, I went on a ride at Six Flags and was kicked off due to my size. That was the most humiliating moment of my life, but I still did nothing to fix it. Three kids later, I packed on even more weight. And my kids wanted me to go on a rollercoaster with them. I refused because I didn't want to re-live that moment again. It was that very moment I realized my weight wasn't just affecting me; it was affecting my entire family. So the following week I started the ketogenic diet. 2 weeks later I was intermittent fasting, with 16:8. Two weeks after that, I started eating only one meal a day with 75% fat, 20%

protein, and 5% carbs. That's when I learned how great of a tool fasting is...especially when eating LCHF. My starting weight was 330 pounds. I'm now 272 pounds– a 58-pound loss. I love my WOE (way of eating) and don't ever plan on stopping–it's a way of life now.

Debbie from Jamaica:

Hi. My Name Is Debbie from Jamaica. I grew up slim, and never had a weight problem in my teens and early twenties. I got a job at 19 in a factory. The pace was fast, and I was moving a lot. I got a promotion and the weight piled on. I was able to shake it off by not eating. The weight went, then I would fall into the routine again, and of course, the weight came on again. I had some stressful work-related issues, so I ended up on Xanax for a short time, probably a month, but it messed me up. I gained weight, and I felt horrible. I tried the lemonade diet and lost a lot of weight, but it did not stay off. I moved from 126 to 160ish. I hated myself.

I went to the gym. Of course, the weight was so slow coming off. Fast forward to 2007. I started University; part-time working while going to school. The weight piled on: snacking in the nights and in class. Reaching home at 11 p.m. and eating again.

I tried hCG injections and lost about twenty pounds, and then I got pregnant in 2012. During the pregnancy, I hardly gained weight. After I had the baby, I was out of control. I gained and gained. I was more depressed. I tried to watch my eating, but nothing worked. I resigned myself to being full of fat. Then came along baby #2. Same story as baby #1.

2016 rolled around. I was 213 pounds. I walked past a mirror and was shocked by my appearance: huge tummy, hump in the back of my neck. I was so sad and felt hopeless. I started to search.

I tried the Daniel diet, and it was so hard. I needed to buy food for myself different from my family, which became a strain on my mind and the budget. I came upon some videos called OMAD Revolution on YouTube. I was impressed at how simple it seemed. He was able to eat regular food, and he lost a lot of weight. I had a glimmer of hope.

I searched on Facebook and came across a wonderful support group. The one meal a day way of life is so stupidly simple, and it works! The last time I checked I lost 18 pounds. I started this in September 2016 as a present to myself. I know I have lost more, but I don't have a working scale. This is so freeing, and I will be eating this way for life. I feel great, and I have a ton of energy. I will not be going back to eating the way I used to. I am sorting out my relationship with food because I used it as a crutch: not happy, eat; angry, eat; happy, celebrate and eat.

Melia K. from San Diego:

I started 16:8, & then moved to 18:6 in October because I felt I could sustain that. I found I was still bingeing, so I looked for something else. One meal a day...that might be the key?

I am now using the 5:2 as my template for a 5:2 OMAD transformation program. (I don't like calling it a DIET.) My calorie intake is 1200:500. My goal is to lose 4 pounds a month for the next year, which will get me to my ideal weight.

As a parent in my 50's with four kids under the age of 20, I want to live longer and be there for them and enjoy them as they continue to grow. Not become a bother to them because of my health issues.

SW: 205 (Oct 27, 2016); CW: 199; GW: 155-145

These programs are great, and the best thing, as I found out... they are interchangeable!

MAKE IT WORK FOR YOU, NOT YOU FOR IT!

Laura from TN:

I am Laura from FL, living in TN for now. I was always too thin until I got married at age 20, then I started to gain weight. I did the yo-yo diet thing, always gaining about 10 pounds extra each time. I gave up trying to lose for a while but then got re-motivated when I went to a concert and almost couldn't fit in the seat. I Googled & stumbled across intermittent fasting. I then discovered one meal a day (OMAD) while researching. I went from 220+ to 150 since March (it is now December). I love it & will eat this way forever. I want to wear a size 8 (I'm in a 14 now), but I am getting there...

Denise from CA:

I tried and tried to make intermittent fasting a part of my life. I, in fact, had been practicing it unbeknownst to me for YEARS in the form of 16:8 when I began to just skip breakfast in order to consume less calories daily. So, when I heard of one meal a day, I thought, great! I thought the 20:4 method should work fine. I started and realized that getting to my weight loss goal I'd need a smaller window for a little bit. 20:4 I believe will be a great maintenance tool. But I was never able to make it past that 19-hour mark. I was ravenous, and I couldn't understand why everyone else was doing it so easily.

After some advice from Gin, fighting it along the way, I finally decided no more Splenda in my coffee and no more artificially sweetened waters. That meant cutting anything with Aspartame in it. I started reading labels and avoiding those products. I didn't think it would make that big a deal, but I knew my body would just thank me for not consuming those poisons anymore.

It was like magic. Not only was I able to go 20 hours without eating, I shortened my eating window to 1.5 hours. It felt incredible! It was like almost overnight. I would say I decided to shorten my window probably five days after stopping the sweeteners, including my beloved Coke Zero. So, there you have it. I'm a believer that those sweeteners spike insulin which causes hunger, not true hunger. I'm so happy I decided to give it a go. In just four days of stopping the sweeteners, I'm down 2 pounds. I think I can live without them!

Katie:

In February of 2014, in anticipation of my 10th Wedding anniversary, I pulled out my wedding gown. I could not even zip it, even with the help of my 9- and 10-year old daughters. There was at least an 8-inch gap between the zippers. I packed the gown back away and vowed that by my 11th anniversary, I would fit back into it. I was 348 pounds.

I started with Atkins which is my old standby. Calorie counting was always an epic failure and left me ravenous and fatter. After the first 20 pounds, I said, "I'm doing this..." Still, I knew that this would not last. I love beans, and lentils, soft fluffy bread, cake. I also had five children and a husband. Eating salmon while they ate beans and rice made me feel guilty.

I stumbled my way through that first 20 pounds, and then I read about JUDDD (Johnson's Up Day/Down Day Diet).

The core problem I had was that I was a binge eater. I grew up in a home where there was no food security. It was feast or famine, so when surrounded with good food, I feasted until I could feast no more. This was a lifelong habit I didn't even realize I had.

JUDDD was awesome for helping me realize the first truth of fasting - hunger wasn't an emergency. I could very well live happily while hungry. It will pass. It doesn't grow and grow.

However, more days then I would like I would find myself binge eating on my "up days." Just eating to eat, stuffing my face to stuff my face. Weight loss was still good...and that saw me through to the 290's. I felt pretty accomplished with a 50-pound weight loss.

At this time, I began trying one meal a day on my "down days." It sometimes worked, but my blood sugar levels would leave me shaking, and dizzy at times. My hormones were all out of whack.

Unexpectedly, I found out I was pregnant with number 6 in 2015. JUDDD was pretty hard to do, so I switched more to a hunger directed eating at that point. But most days I just ate what I wanted without overdoing it. By the end of the pregnancy and postpartum period in January of 2016, I weighed right back in the 290's.

At that point, I decided to switch more to the one meal a day eating style. I had had an emotional breakthrough that I was a binge eater. That's the why of it. How my relationship with food was messed up. No diet would ever be successful if I didn't figure that out. I did a lot of emotional work while pregnant.

My blood sugar levels made one meal a day very hard at first. I would shake, and feel nauseous, grumpy, and dizzy. Sometimes while preparing my family's lunch, I would say, "Oh, I can't do this!" and eat, feeling more terrible with each bite.

At first, to get me through those tough first couple of weeks, I would allow myself hard boiled eggs when the worst of the spells would hit. Not having to suffer through the shakes made it possible because I was comfortable. That is how it became a lifestyle for me.

Eventually, I didn't need the eggs one day. Things began to be corrected in my body. I have been doing one meal a day fasting on either 18:6 schedule or 23:1 since. I have days where I wake up hungry, and it feels like a different hunger, and I eat those days. The next day I am back on. Sure, I take my breaks also. The longest has been for two months, and wow. I felt like crap after that long of an absence.

Still, when I came back to it - I didn't need the eggs this time, or anything. It was like riding a bicycle. My body knew what to do.

As of today, I am at a 116 pounds loss, and if I didn't count the year I took off for pregnancy and postpartum - it would have taken me probably about a year to 16 months to lose that. Wonderful results for being able to eat what you want, for curing hormone issues, and for people on a budget who can't afford specific foods needed for a diet.

One meal a day has saved me. I have no doubt the 70 pounds extra I am carrying will come off this year.

By the way, my wedding gown fit by my 11th wedding anniversary just as it did on my wedding day. Now it is too loose.

Sandy, from Port Huron, MI:
I'm 63 now. I was always a big girl. 183 when I graduated high school. Dieted all my adult life. About a year and a half ago I found Dr. Bert Herring and Fast 5. And lost 30 pounds. And then I found this great group…One Meal a Day (OMAD), and switched over to this to get the last 10 pounds off.

I love this way of eating. I will do it for the rest of my life. I'm 150 now at 5' 6". I'M HAPPY WEARING SIZE MEDIUM, instead of 1X.

Mari:

I have *The Obesity Code* book. I've been high fat/keto for ten days. I have a weight loss goal. I maintained a 50-pound loss (portion control, 19:5, bite counting, low carb off & on) for 16 months doing one meal a day (OMAD). I did gain some weight over the holidays this time last year, but lost it all very quickly upon returning to OMAD. Since October 2, I'm down another 30 pounds doing 19:5 or 23:1 & bite counting. I still have 55 pounds to lose to reach my goal of BMI 21, which is where I was when I was dating my husband 22 years ago. I'm wearing clothes I haven't fit into since 2008. I've done 2 7-day water fasts (in July of 2014 & again at the end of this past September), and plan to do so for the next seven days, starting noon today. This is a reminder to myself & any doubters that this works.

Pam from Toronto, age 42:

I follow this way of eating for health issues, specifically digestive issues. I've spent the last four years trying to get rid of small intestinal bacterial overgrowth (found in 80% of people with IBS). I saw two regular MD's, three gastroenterologists, and five naturopaths. I spent thousands of dollars and had numerous tests done, and was given herbs, supplements, prescriptions, etc. Every time I ate, I would get symptoms of discomfort and lower belly distension. I developed a fear of eating. Last June, I had a tummy bug and couldn't eat most of the day, but made myself eat something at night, as I didn't want to lose weight. I did this for four days and noticed I had zero digestive issues during this time. I researched and found the warrior diet and then the one meal a day (OMAD) Facebook group. I haven't had any digestive issues since OMAD. I am thrilled, and my doctor supports this WOE (way of eating) and said fasting is the best thing I can do for longevity. I'm so happy.

Rebecca:

I have tended to be overweight my whole life. I remember when it started. I was around six or seven years old and came home from school and felt hungry so I ate a snack. I must have been exceptionally hungry that day because it felt sooo amazing to eat that snack! At the wise age of six, I then rationalized that snacks made you feel better. So it began. My weight has yo-yoed ever since then. I have tried almost every mainstream diet out there. Low carb, even keto. Low calorie. Low fat. Several small meals. These diets work temporarily, but I can never stick to them. I have no willpower. About two months ago the dawn hit me.... Back when I was a smoker, I never ate breakfast and lunch. Not intentionally, I just took my breaks and lunch at work outside to smoke and never ate. That was my thinnest during my adult life. When I quit smoking and subsequently started eating three meals a day, I gained roughly 70 pounds. That brings me to present day, and the dawn that came to me was one meal a day. I Googled the phrase and realized it is something that people actually do! I found the Facebook group and started right away. I am currently around two months in and have lost 13 pounds. To some, that may seem slow, but let me point out that I eat whatever I want during my one-to-two-hour window. Anything... And all of it that I want. That's what I love about this way of eating. I have eaten half of a large pepperoni pizza a few times. Half of a dinner box from McDonald's. I eat fast food. Restaurant food. And dessert every single day. I know that eating healthier would increase my weight loss speed, and I see that I have started to crave healthy foods as well. I think I will slowly work my way to healthier foods, but for right now this is working, and the freedom to eat whatever I want is letting me stick to it like I never could with standard "diets." I can't wait to see what lies ahead for me with this lifestyle.

SA, from Soweto/Meadowlands:
I've tried everything, anything, spent money, but since I started eating one meal a day in August, I look and feel good about myself. I used to weigh 80 kilograms, and now I'm 69 kilograms. My ideal weight is 65 kilograms.

My big belly is gone, and even my skin is beautiful. What makes my life more exciting is that I'm from size 40 to 34.

When people ask I tell them. Their response—shame, food is so good! At times I end up not eating but make a fruit smoothie. I drink lots of water. Also, before bedtime, I drink warm ginger water and 1st thing in the morning I drink plain warm water. You'll be amazed with the morning water and what it does to your body.

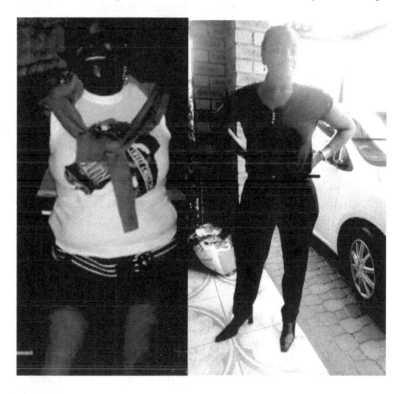

JJ from Maine:
Here's my story. I did not embark on fasting for weight loss, though losing a few pounds was going to be a side benefit. I started fasting as I saw an article that said fasting would decrease inflammation in the body. I had already been doing 12-hour fasts for the last few years, so thought I would escalate it and do 16-18 hours. Back in 2003, I was diagnosed with an uncommon form of arthritis that affects my spine. The doctors were telling

me I needed to get on an injectable to keep my spine from fusing. So, this summer in July, I took an injectable drug, and it stays in the blood/body for 30 days. Well, I had pain relief, but I also had an uncommon reaction in that it affected my neurological system and it was like I was high for 30 days. It affected my reading and writing. I just did not care about anything, and I was really happy… like 15 out of 10. So needless to say, I was not going to do that again. I prayed for God to show me something to do, and then the article came along. I only intended to fast on, say, Monday, Wednesday, and Friday, but I was on vacation, and it morphed into 18-hour days for three days in a row. It was at that point that I noticed I had no pain in my knees and I had a lot of energy. So I went another day, no pain in my shoulder. Another day, no pain in my back. Weird. So I just kept going. Then it occurred to me that I felt like I did on the medication, but not so escalated…just a 10 out of 10 for happiness. I felt very peaceful and mellow and had so much energy. In the middle of October, I thought, gee, I might hurt myself if I keep this up (as all my friends and family thought it couldn't be healthy) so I went back to eating normally. By day three, I could not get out of bed… Soooo much back pain. Unreal. Could not figure out what happened. Next morning, went back to fasting, and three days later the pain was gone…kept it up until Thanksgiving. Only intended to go off fasting for the holiday ("free range eating"), but it expanded to five days. By Wednesday, I was in pain and couldn't walk around. Back on the fasting… 100% pain relief. Even today, in 15-degree weather: no pain. Mind blown. Still trying to get a hold of my doctor in Boston to see if we can somehow test blood inflammatory states to see if this is able to be seen on tests, but just having no pain is unreal for me. Pain has been my prison for most of my life. The last month or two has been a true life-changer. The added bonus of losing some weight and my IBS (irritable symptoms) subsiding is another plus. I thank God every day for giving me an answer and providing healing. Thank you so much for reading my story.

Katie C.:

I have always been on the chunky side as far back as I can remember. Had four kids and was at my highest weight at 210. I have tried every diet pill that you can name; tried them all. I would lose a bit and then reward myself with a treat. I was in a stressful time in my life and working in a restaurant and just could not eat the food anymore, so now when I look back, I guess I was fasting without knowing it. I lost all my weight and was at my lowest weight ever at 135 pounds. My life got better and stress-free. I felt great. My sisters kept asking me what I was using to lose my weight, and I told them I was not using anything at the time. They then wanted to know what I was eating. I told them that I only eat dinner, don't like breakfast, and did not have time for lunch at work. I was told over and over that I was very unhealthy, that I needed my 3+ meals a day at my age. And so it began, eating 3 meals plus, and before I knew what happened I was back at 190 pounds with arthritis in my back and hands, and a bloated stomach to the point I could not breathe. Many, many tests, and nothing showed up. My knees got so bad that when I was on the floor playing with the grandkids, I could not get up without holding on for support. Sleeping all night was a joke. I would sleep 3 hours a night, get up in the morning and just want to cry (and did many times) as I was so tired. Went to see my doctor and was put on meds for sleep, but still was awake till 3 a.m., so I tossed them in the trash.

I went to see the kids in Calgary for Thanksgiving and was shocked at the weight my son and daughter-in-law had lost, and she said it was not just the weight loss that was good, but she had also dropped all her meds for diabetes. I returned home and started my search. I came across one meal a day (OMAD) and started August 13, 2016. I am down 30-some pounds, and inches keep falling off. But best of all is I now remember again what a full night's sleep feels like and my arthritis is gone. I can breathe without difficulty, my stomach bloat is gone, and

151

the ulcer meds I have been on, I no longer need. Looking back now, I was fasting when I lost all my weight and did not know it was a way of life. I am 58 years and plan on being around for my 17 grandchildren for a few more years. I love the freedom I have now with OMAD.
I only wish I could go back and get refunded for all the money I wasted on gimmicks.

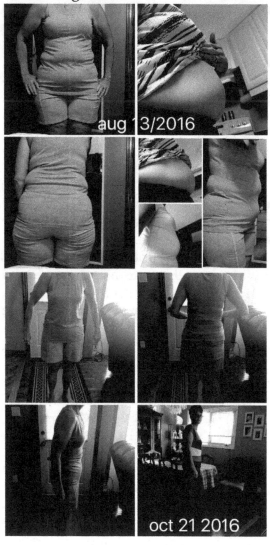

Jen:

I need to share some excitement - OMAD is working and feels comfortable and better than anything I've tried. The scale is moving slowly, but the biggest change I've seen with this way of eating (WOE) is eliminating my binging. A day for me used to look like this: pre-plan and re-plan my food for the day, trying to stay under my calorie allotment. Think about food ALL DAY because I was denying myself what I liked and picking foods to stay within my goal. Because of lunch, my dinner would be smaller, and by the time I got my kids in bed, I would be hungry again. Because I can't fall asleep on an empty stomach, I would deny myself more food, and then say forget it and raid the cupboards. I would go to bed full but wake up frustrated at myself and the scale never moved. Every single day.

Now I feel slight hunger during the day, but it's manageable, and I eat whatever I want for dinner. Yesterday I had a long day and came home and made myself everything I wanted: breaded chicken, potato wedges, cheese balls, and jalapeño poppers. Totaled it up in my head, and it was still less than I used to eat with the nightly cupboard raids. I go to bed full and satisfied now and the bit of hunger in the day is nothing compared to my insatiable appetite I used to have before bed. This is amazing. I finally feel in control, I'm not counting calories which (was ruling my life) and I'm eating what I actually want vs. what fits into lunch and dinner calorie goals. This is what I've needed all along!

Anna Ball from TN:

I'm 23 years old, and 5'8". I have been doing intermittent fasting for 9 months. Picture on the left was 3/24/16. Picture on the right was 11/13/16. I have lost 52 pounds.

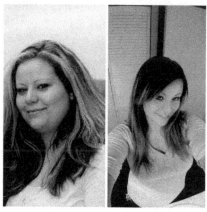

I went from a size 16-18 to a size 10-12 depending on who makes the pants. I went from an XXL to a large. My weight gain started after I got pregnant and continued after pregnancy. I tried counting calories and eating healthy. I lost a few pounds but didn't keep it off. I did the military diet for the three days, but I did not lose a pound. I did the Dolly Parton diet (soup cleanse), and I didn't lose any weight. I started intermittent fasting at my heaviest: 232 pounds. I started on the 5bd (5 bite diet), which made me feel horrible, weak, and tired. I lost some weight, but it was very hard. As I was looking for more information about the 5bd I ran across "one meal a day," or OMAD. I thought, "That sounds more realistic and sustainable." I have been on OMAD for 8 months now. I feel amazing and energized. Before OMAD I was always so tired, even after waking up. My depression and anxiety have improved as well. OMAD has changed my life, not just my weight. But I have this need to improve everything else around me too. I have even organized all the closets in the house… Lol.

What's my routine? What do I drink? How long is my window? I wake up, and drink black coffee until 1 p.m.

Then I drink water, water with lemon, ice tea, or water w/lemon and a little salt. Then I eat dinner sometime after 4 p.m. Depends on when it's done or when I get hungry. I have a window normally no longer than 3 hours. And sometimes I do eat lunch for my one meal.

What do I eat? Do I eat carbs or low carb? I eat whatever I want. I really do. I eat until SATISFIED not stuffed or sick. I go out to eat once a week. I eat carbs. But I do have days when I watch my carbs (bread/flour and sweets) and try to keep them kinda low.

Any food/drink that I avoid in my window? Not really... I eat anything I want. BUT, I don't drink any type of soda. Makes me feel bloated.

How did I start OMAD? I woke up and had black coffee and water until dinner. I was super busy that day. So I didn't have time to think about food.

Did I work out? No, I did not. I am now because I want to build a little lean muscle and tone up.

Final words from Gin

As you see, intermittent fasting is changing lives. It's time for YOU to make the commitment to changing YOURS. I look forward to seeing you around, maybe in one of our Facebook groups. I can't wait to read YOUR success story! Please make sure to share it with us.